Racialization of Coronavirus and Hate Crimes

Racialization of Coronavirus and Hate Crimes

Written by Austin Mardon, Fatima Arshad Syed,
Faried Nasir, and Catherine Mardon

Designed by Ethan Gabriel Saldana

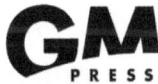

GM PRESS

2020

A Golden Meteorite Press Book
Printed in Canada

Copyright © 2020 by Austin Mardon, Fatima Arshad Syed, Faried Nasir, Catherine Mardon, Ethan Gabriel Saldana

First Printing: 2020

ISBN 978-1-77369-152-7

Golden Meteorite Press
103 11919 82 St NW
Edmonton, AB T5B 2W3
www.goldenmeteoritepress.com

We acknowledge the support of Canada Service Corps, TakingITGlobal, and the Government of Canada in promotional materials associated with the Project.

Thank you.

Table of Contents

Chapter 1: Introduction to COVID-19 Racialization of Coronavirus and Hate Crimes

COVID-19 has taken the world by storm. Heavily contagious and spreading rapidly, the virus is easily able to be transmitted from one person to another. The virus is part of the coronavirus family which are usually found in animals. However, in the case of humans, coronaviruses can be a greater threat. Some other examples of coronaviruses are Severe Acute Respiratory Syndrome (SARS) as well as the Middle East Respiratory Syndrome (MERS) ("Q&A on Coronaviruses", 2020). The COVID-19 virus' usual symptoms are "fever, dry cough, and tiredness". Most recover from the virus, however about 1 in 5 people who get the virus can become severely ill ("Q&A on Coronaviruses", 2020). These people are usually those with pre-existing conditions such as high blood pressure, diabetes, or cancer. But these symptoms are not exclusive to these people. The elderly also are at a higher risk of severe illness from the virus ("Q&A on Coronaviruses", 2020). Moreover, a variety of different types of otherwise healthy people have become seriously ill because of the virus' effects. Added to this, the virus spreads very easily. This is done through sneezing, speaking, and coughing in the presence of those not infected—making it very easy to transmit the virus if one is not wearing a facemask ("Q&A on Coronaviruses", 2020).

Based on this, it becomes clear why so many precautions are being taken to prevent the virus from spreading to more people by governments around the world. Many nations have declared a state of emergency amid the rapidly changing situation. Whole countries have shut down seemingly overnight. People around the world have been forced to take precautions to protect themselves and their loved ones from the virus. Many have been forced to leave their jobs; being laid off and taking government assistance to survive. This has led the economy to take a toll, with many restaurants and places of work closing entirely

("Q&A on Coronaviruses", 2020). Other workplaces such as retail and service industries have also been affected. Others who are considered "essential" have been allowed to continue working—but also risk their lives as well as those around them to do so. This rapid change and the relative novelty of the virus has left us as a global community confused.

Many have developed strong fears about the virus and what the future holds. Due to social distancing practices and isolation many of us have remained indoors and have had very little social interactions. The pandemic has become the focus of the news. This has led some outlets to take this as an opportunity to release information without checking their facts. In some specific cases, false information is being released to push an agenda that validates false information. This may lead us to gathering information from the internet and looking for specific groups to blame as it pertains to the creation and transmission of the virus. Yet, this information may not always be correct. Moreover, often, social media platforms are being used to spread false information relating to COVID-19 that is motivated which in turn is spread even more rapidly through confirmation bias—the belief that one's own prejudices are true, leading them to seek out information that validates their biased beliefs (Heshmat, 2015). This has led specific minority groups such as Asian minorities to be targeted. To understand why, we must first understand the concept of racialization.

What is racialization?

To define racialization, we must first define race. The term is difficult to define as it implies a concept of "racial purity". It is an abstract term with no biological meaning. Sociologically speaking however, it is a different story. Certain assumptions are the basis of this idea. The first is that it is socially constructed. This means that society has set up the terms to define race implicitly (Foster, 2006). The second is that it depends on the "time and space". What this means is that the concept of race will differ depending on what time-period you live in (Foster, 2006). Moreover, the location on the Earth in which you reside also plays a role in one's notion of what race is. The third quality used to define race is that these previously mentioned factors play a role and are "attached with status" and meaning (Foster, 2006). This means that the different socialized races each bring meaning into their supposed race based on the definition which society gives them. While it may be

2

a "biological myth" to define race, it is a "social reality". This means that the consequences of having different races are real. Misinterpretations of this concept is common. The largest falsehood in this sense is that the concept of race does not change. The concept is often referred to as something that is set in stone—rather than something that has various meanings across different cultures and historical frames (Foster, 2006). They are related to identity and personhood rather than biology.

Now, when it comes to racialization—in this book we are referring to the concept of "the racialized other". This refers to the hierarchy that is often developed within cultures when referring to race (Foster, 2006). Some races are deemed superior while others are deemed inferior. The whole notion includes ideas of power where one race can subjugate other races into controlling them. Exclusion and inclusion in this idea is all based in the idea of race. Based on this, racialization refers to singling out specific groups for "real or imagined physical characteristics" (Foster, 2006). We prescribe certain connotations to specific races based on conditions that are unique to each culture. There becomes those who fit within the condition to not be excluded while others fall outside that realm based on criteria designed to exclude.

Racialization then expands into stigmatization. This is the "mark of disgrace" (Foster, 2006). Individuals are cast out and isolated by their social group. They are deemed "too different" to be considered part of the group. They do not have social acceptance. As a result, not only do they miss out on social interaction but also on material opportunities that arise with it. This leads to marginalization—when stigmatization leads specific groups to not have access to the same socio-economic, cultural, and political benefits which society offers (Foster, 2006). While these definitions do not offer the origin of these distinctions, it becomes clear that the subversion of power plays a role in how they are defined. Those who are not in the majority in terms of their supposed "racial" makeup, therefore fall into being defined as "the racialized other" (Foster, 2006). In terms of COVID-19, in North America, this "mark of disgrace" has sadly been given to Asian minorities.

Discrimination of Asians around the Globe

Asian minorities are being targeted because of the virus' origins in China. What this has led to is powerful individuals around the world condemning them for reasons they have no control over. Leaders from many western nations have come out against Asian communities because of xenophobic anti-Chinese ideas. These countries include individuals from the US, UK, Italy, Spain, Greece, France, and Germany ("Covid-19 Fueling Anti-Asian Racism", 2020). They are fueling a rhetoric that allows for xenophobic conspiracy theories to thrive. Some examples of this practice have been made public. President Trump's continued use of the term "Chinese virus" has allowed for Asian communities within the US to become vulnerable to blame for the virus ("Covid-19 Fueling Anti-Asian Racism", 2020).

He has created an environment where it is okay to discriminate against people based on their race. Blame extends beyond the US as well. The governor of the Veneto region of Italy offered that Italians were better suited to deal with the virus because they have been "culturally strong to hygiene…whereas…the Chinese [eat] mice alive" ("Covid-19 Fueling Anti-Asian Racism", 2020). While he did later apologize for the statement, in his position, it becomes easy to see why this anti-Chinese rhetoric is spreading throughout the Western world. Other claims have been even more outlandish. The Education Minister of Brazil offered the idea that this pandemic was a way for the Chinese government's "plan for world domination" ("Covid-19 Fueling Anti-Asian Racism", 2020).

Quotes like this have led to an increase in racist attacks against Asians around the world. The likes of which are not limited to "beatings, violent bullying, threats, racist abuse, and discrimination". In Italy alone, the number of reported crimes against Asians has been 50—with numbers still on the rise. Other countries around the world are seeing similar attacks against their Asian communities. From taunting to racialized violence, from Africa to Australia, the number of cases against Asian workers has only risen. The situation does not change in Canada. In a recent poll, 1 in 5 Canadians felt unsafe next to "an Asian person on the bus" ("Understanding the Impact of COVID-19", 2020). What this shows is the lack of awareness about the cause of the virus and how the virus has been racialized even though there is no scientific backing behind these ideas. Instead, xenophobic tendencies have risen out of fear and anxiety for the virus (Kang, 2020). Based on this, this book aims to deconstruct the racialization of the virus while also exploring the history of hate crimes to gain a better understanding for our current predicament.

Outline

Now, I will offer an outline of what this book aims to present. We will begin by offering an account of the myths around COVID-19. This will include the various conspiracy theories related to the virus and its association with China. Then, there will be an attempt to resolve these conspiracies through an analysis of the virus itself. Following this, there will be an account of the various hate crimes which have a history within North America as they pertain to race. This will allow a point of comparison to COVID-19. After this, there will be a historical survey of racialized disease. This will further allow us to use history to understand our current situation more effectively. Then, there will be a shift of focus towards the current racialized violence occurring against Asians around the globe. There will be a survey of the current trends of racism provided. Afterwards, there will be another shift of focus towards concepts related to race such as fears, stereotypes and propaganda as it pertains to the virus. These chapters aim to put racialized anxiety to rest buy showing that the recent trend of bigotry is the result of misconstrued ideas that have been perpetuated by xenophobic social media posts not only buy hate groups but buy actual politicians themselves. The fear of the country of China also plays a role in this racialized violence. Any biases individuals have towards the country itself manifests itself towards Chinese individuals. Lastly, this book will end by providing an account of ways individuals can go about preventing hate crimes.

Chapter 2: Eugenics and Biowarfare: The Myths and Realities of COVID-19

The current COVID-19 pandemic has led to various myths about the virus' origins making it difficult to differentiate reality from fiction. Through the advent of dubious online news outlets and social media, false ideas about the virus have been spread rapidly. From use as a Chinese bioweapon to blame being tossed around to specific groups, the virus is brimming with controversy. Additionally, the spread of the virus has brought archaic ideas to light and made them more widespread—namely in relation to scientific racism (Jones, 2020). The virus disproportionally affects the elderly as well as those with pre-existing conditions while the mortality rate for other groups falls quite low (Jones, 2020).

In relation to this, there have been a plethora of attacks against these groups calling for their "sacrifice" in order to allow the rest of the world to return to normal (Jones, 2020). Moreover, the controversy extends to an almost tribalist ground with one French doctor calling for testing for a vaccine to be done on Africans to push past the animal testing portion of the vaccine trials (Jones, 2020). In North America, we are seeing a decline in the sales of Chinese restaurant sales disproportionately from other types of cuisine. In some areas of the United States they are down "at least 70 percent" (Heil and Carman, 2020). What all these examples show is a new set of xenophobic attitudes which are surfacing during the pandemic. This chapter will attempt to highlight two specific issues related to COVID-19. These include the ideas of eugenics and biowarfare. The reach of these attitudes ranges from a fear of anything Chinese due to the virus' origins within the city of Wuhan and go as far as calling for the death of the elderly. Yet, Chinese food vendors living in the United States are not responsible for the virus. Nor do the elderly have any reason to die so that others can shop without masks or go to restaurants. So where do these new xenophobic attitudes originate from? To answer this question, we must differentiate fact from fake news.

Biowarfare and COVID-19

Let us begin by looking at some powerful misconceptions about the virus. The idea of biowarfare is a consistent theme when it comes to the discussion of COVID-19. Biowarfare is the utilization of pathogens such as bacteria or viruses by nations. These countries use them to destroy their enemies through deadly infection. In this context, misleading claims suggest that the COVID-19 virus was created by the Chinese government as a bioweapon. The origins of these claims' stems from the fact that the virus is so new that it is difficult for scientists to offer research that negates these speculative ideas. Furthermore, the idea that COVID-19 is a bioweapon was spread unknowingly through social media platforms instilling the idea that it is a bioweapon in people's minds. All these claims are unfounded and have spread not by experts but instead by those in power.

For example, politicians have offered their own ideas on this "so-called" Chinese conspiracy which led to the creation of the virus. US Senator Tom Cotton offered in a tweet that while not personally knowing the origin of the virus that the city of Wuhan has a superlab which "works with the world's most deadly pathogens to include…coronavirus" (Lee, 2020). Even journalists have become vocal about their fear of a Chinese pathogen. New York Post writer Steve Mosher wrote an article titled "Don't buy China's story: The coronavirus may have leaked from a lab" (Lee, 2020). Yet, neither of these claims indicate guilt. There are a variety of different types of coronaviruses so implying that one specific strain was released into a nation's own people would be illogical.

Moreover, Steve Mosher is also the writer of a book titled "Bully of Asia: Why China's 'Dream' Is the New Threat to the World Order" (Lee, 2020). Having read these titles, one gains insight into the motivations of individuals who spread this fear mongering. There is a heavy bias at play. It is a fear of the Chinese which is fueling these ideas, not any scientific evidence which suggests this specific strain of coronavirus was artificially created (Kaszeta, 2020). On the other hand, scientists have not found any evidence to suggest that this virus was created by humans—or that the Chinese government created the bug to destroy their western allies. The claim is false and in commenting on this issue the WHO director general Tedros Adhanom Ghebreyesus offered that "fake news spreads faster" than the virus itself (Carbarnaro, 2020). This leads me to the next issue which the virus has brought to light. The use of COVID-19 by the Chinese government as a biological weapon is a failed idea because the coronavirus has also infected millions of Chinese people themselves. It makes no sense for a nation to infect their own people. Added to this fact, there is no benefit to this agent being used for war by any group.

To back up this idea, scientists have been able to verify that the virus originates in bat populations—not in human laboratories. They claim that "RNA sequences" of COVID-19 "are like those "that silently circulate in bats" (Lee, 2020). This implies the origin of the virus is not man-made and demonstrates that the fear mongering for the Chinese that has been developed is unjustified. It also demonstrates that the virus was not made "accidentally" by the Chinese lab and then released onto the population of Wuhan (Lee, 2020). Moreover, a similar study focused on the analysis of genetic sequences offered that the virus clings onto human cells systematically and destroys them. While it may seem like it was a targeted attempt to destroy other humans, the reality is our current technology cannot produce such specific results. Therefore, the virus must have developed naturally from the transmission of bats. The bats then interacted with some third-party animal which has not yet been deduced. This animal was then sold in a Wuhan wet-market in China. These markets are often crowded and create a breeding ground for viruses to spread easily. Another fact that refutes the claim that COVID-19 is a bioweapon is that the rate of death is so low. If this were in fact designed to kill other humans, why would it have such a low death rate? —with some estimates ranging from 1% to 3.4% (Lee, 2020).

Eugenics and COVID-19

Now, let us turn attention to the rise of eugenic attitudes due to coronaviruses. Eugenics is the belief that some groups are "biologically "better" than others" (Shanks, 2020). Proponents of this belief offer that their pseudoscientific ideals should drive the socio-political landscape. The ideas are not new dating back as far as Plato (Shanks, 2020). In its current form the eugenics movement can trace its lineage in the late

19th century within Britain (Shanks, 2020). During this time, Social Darwinist attitudes were taking root within the western world leading to prospects such as colonialism. Later, western nations have had a history of sterilising individuals with mental illness as late as the 1920s (Shanks, 2020). Only after the atrocities of Nazi Germany in World War II did the movement finally become obsolete (Shanks, 2020).

But the pandemic has brought the idea of eugenics back to mainstream attention. The virus disproportionally affects specific ethnic groups as well those with disabilities. In a statement, the director of Tuskegee University's National Centre for Bioethics in Research and Healthcare offered that he was "not surprised" by this rise (Shanks, 2020). In fact, he believes that politicians did not collect ethnic data about the virus because "they knew what data would tell them". This in the United States refers to the fact that black lives are affected disproportionately higher than any other groups by COVID-19. This problem has implications outside of the United States and Canada. For example, in India, a Hindu majority state the New York Times offers that "officials are blaming an Islamic group for spreading the virus". In Singapore, migrant workers have been "packed into unsanitary dormitories". In China, African migrant workers "are being demonised" over the virus. What the virus has done is to normalize fear of the "other". In all countries, we are employing archaic attitudes by using the weak as scapegoats.

Other scapegoats are the old—as I mentioned previously. For example, when asked about the economy in relation to COVID-19 the lieutenant governor of Texas offered that it might be time "to ask whether the nation might be better off letting a few hundred thousand people die" (Jones, 2020). Attitudes like this present a common and dangerous sentiment. Individuals are dividing others into groups. Those who deserve to live, and those who deserve to die. But my own argument against this mentality, is that while the risk is low against coronavirus in the average person—there is still a relatively low chance of death. If someone told me to go outside into a group of a million infected people, and that there was a 3% of dying I would flat out refuse. I think any rational person would do the same. So why then should we have to not only sacrifice the elderly and those with disabilities? —and ourselves on top of that for what is a little payoff if it can be prevented in our highly developed nation with social safety nets.

Moreover, the truth of the matter gets more complicated than just referring to ethnicity. What it really comes down to is another factor of eugenics—class (Dodds and Karlsen, 2020). Those on the lower rungs of the socio-economic ladder are more likely to get infected because they are often deemed "essential". For example, those working at meatpacking plants were still required to work under the lockdown within the United States (Dodds and Karlsen, 2020). This means that these lower socio-economic groups are more likely to get infected because they must continue working and interacting within the outside world. They do not get the benefits of leaving work and taking care of their health. They are deemed expendable through policies which do not allow them to leave work. Then, when they contract the virus it spreads to their homes which are often overcrowded as well. This idea is backed by a study done at the University of Bristol in the UK. Researchers found that the virus affects Bangladeshi individuals twice as much, Pakistani people three times as much and Black Africans four times as much as their white British counterparts (Dodds and Karlsen, 2020). The study offers that individuals often assume the odds of contracting the virus is the result of genetic "predispositions" or some strange cultural behavior which causes this (Dodds and Karlsen, 2020). Yet, the authors of the study argue that these assumptions are false as they are based on the idea that individuals across specific ethnicities, religions or cultures all behave in similar ways (Dodds and Karlsen, 2020). Other false ideas which the study contests is a link between certain vitamin deficiencies or common diseases to the rise of COVID-19 among certain ethnic groups. These are also not likely the reason these groups have this high rate of the virus. Instead, the real reason comes down to the socioeconomic factors. The ethnic groups which are affected disproportionately by the virus are the same ones who are living "in overcrowded accommodation" as a result of a lack of "financial safety nets" (Dodds and Karlsen, 2020). They are forced to work or die. They are therefore more likely to get the virus and spread it to those in their surroundings. The researchers also found that these same groups also are less likely to have full time employment or be poorly paid compared to their white British counterparts. They are forced to work during the pandemic leaving more and more opportunities for them to be affected by the virus.

Conclusion: What does it all mean?

The discussed controversies surrounding COVID-19 demonstrate a mentality towards fear. Ultimately, this situation is showing us just how cruel we can be towards those who are different. This does not only apply within a North American context, but across the world as well. The myths that have formed around the virus are nothing new. They are the same archaic ideas which have driven humans against each other for thousands of years. Yet, the difference now is that it is becoming increasingly easy to see why those individuals in power spread propaganda related to the virus. The reality of the situation is ultimately that responsibility in this topic is a tricky situation. More so than that, there can be no accountability on the global level because the cause of the virus is natural, not man made in a lab, like some would have you believe. With this idea in mind, we can move forward together as a global community by taking action to prevent the spread of the virus instead of spreading hatred.

Chapter 3: Hate Crimes and Why They Are Still Relevant Today

Recently, a video leaked of a Calgary man spitting on an Asian minority while she was minding her own business in a local park. This is part of a new wave of hate crimes against Asian minorities within the Western world (Ahrens et al, 2020). As established in the previous chapter, this rise is unjustified and based in scapegoating towards minorities. But is this pattern new? Or is a historical trend of placing the blame against ethnic minorities? Hate crimes against minorities is an idea that dates to early human history. From Roman prosecution of Christians to Nazi concentration camps, the topic of hate crimes against minority groups has examples that sadly find their place in many cultures throughout the world. What this chapter intends to do is to provide a general overview of hate crimes against ethnic minorities within North America. These crimes are not always motivated through the rise of disease but always follow xenophobic reasoning. Therefore, this analysis will serve to further illustrate the socio-culture fears that have arisen during the COVID-19 crisis.

What is a Hate crime?

A hate crime is a hard term to define. It is a very general term that can describe the intentional use of abuse towards a victim who meets some specific "characteristic" which the offender dislikes ("Disproportionate Harm", 2015). The definition becomes more and more difficult to define past that point. This is due to a variety of reasons. According to the Government of Canada, there "has been little systematic research" on the topic ("Disproportionate Harm", 2015). This makes it difficult to correlate how frequent cases of abuse can be. This has led to different organizations using different terms to define the term. For example, the Toronto Metropolitan Police uses the term to refer to crimes which are "based solely upon the victim's race, religion, nationality, ethnic origin, sexual orientation...or disability" ("Disproportionate Harm", 2015). Others define the term as simply being motivated based on bias. Taken together, we can see that the idea of hate crimes is based in difference. If individuals deem that others are different in specific ways, they will create nonsensical truths about them with no logical backing—leading them to commit crimes against them. This essay will focus specifically on the ethnic and cultural biases that individuals create which I will now discuss in the form of case studies.

Case Studies

African Americans

The history of hate crimes towards African Americans in the United States follows closely to the ending of legal slavery within the United States. Around the late 1800s, white Americans in the Southern United States began blaming many of their economic issues on the newly freed slaves in the area. They had lost their main source of income and used the African American population as a scapegoat for the issues they were facing. The main way their bigotry was expressed was through lynching. A lynch mob is a group of people who kill an individual for a supposed crime without any trial (Lartey and Morris, 2018). They were used to "terrorize black Americans into submission" ("History of Lynchings, 2020). The torture individuals endured went beyond just being hanged. They would be burned and "mob members would take pieces of their flesh and bone as souvenirs". In some cases, their actions would result in law enforcement joining them even without any legal precedent. The most popular states they would take place in were Mississippi, Florida, Arkansas, Georgia, and Louisiana had the highest rate of lynchings overall.

Furthermore, the groups which were part of lynchings demonstrates the way hate crime was ingrained into the minds of white Americans. It was mostly not seen as a way of maintaining a power hierarchy-but rather a "joyous moment of wholesome celebration" (Lartey and Morris, 2018). Families would come with even their "youngest children". A 1930 editorial from the Raleigh News offered that men would joke "loudly at the sight of the bleeding body". Moreover, young girls would giggle at the sight of the "blood that dripped from the Negro's nose" (Lartey and Morris, 2018). These suggest the dehumanizing which lynching of African Americans had. Furthermore, the taking of "souvenirs" made the hate crime appear as if it were some game and they were taking a prize.

Yet, this was not a "rare" occasion when the lynchings would occur. Statistics suggest that between 1882 and 1968, 4743 lynchings were reported ("History of Lynchings, 2020). Over 70 percent of these lynchings occurred to Black Americans. The real number is likely larger than this figure as many of the lynchings during this time went unreported ("History of Lynchings, 2020). While the underlying reason for lynching was rooted in racism, the justification for the hate crime was given alternative reasons. The people committing the hate crimes offered that they were protecting "white women" or were punishing those that committed homicides. Yet, the number of lynchings was disproportionately affecting black individuals—demonstrating that the crime was racially motivated ("History of Lynchings, 2020).

Latin Americans

Like African Americans, hate crimes against Latinos in the United States is still an ongoing issue with over 485 reported cases in 2018 alone (Hassan, 2009). While its history is often overlooked there are many incidences of hate crimes against Latin Americans. Texas is a hotbed for controversy relating to hate crimes against Latin Americans. In the late 1900s many instances occurred which aimed to create "white economic control" within the state. After the US-Mexico War in 1848, many Anglo Americans settled on the new territory. But this led to the displacement of indigenous Americans who had been living the land for generations (Mosley, 2019). Moreover, Mexican landowners in the region were also displaced. To justify this displacement, Mexicans were often "portrayed as bandits" who stole the land (Mosley, 2019). But it was just a tool to garner economic disparity and place white Americans on a higher plane than their Mexican counterparts.

Another example of hate crime towards Latinos within Texas can be seen in the Porvenir massacre of 1918. This event took place in the area around El Paso, Texas. A group of Texas Rangers, "the state police" of the area, joined a group of supposed "vigilantes" and surrounded the

Mexican majority city of Porvenir, Texas (Mosley, 2019). The killing resulted in the death of 15 men as well as some children. No one was prosecuted and because the state police were involved it demonstrates that injustice done against Latino minorities have been allowed to occur legally within the history of the United States. There was no reason given for these killings but the city itself was just a ranching town (Mosley, 2019). This demonstrates the lack of justification used in some instances of hate crimes. These two examples demonstrate a pattern of anti-immigrant and anti-Mexican attitudes which became justified through law enforcement. Later history suggests that like Jim Crow laws for African Americans, similar policies were designed to segregate Mexican Americans. These forced sterilization laws and anti-voting legislation along with celebrated militarization of the border to keep out Mexicans (Iturralde, 2009).

Jewish Minorities

It may surprise you that hate crimes against Jewish people have reached an all-time high last year (Lazarus, 2019). With over 2107 hate crimes committed last year; the number surpassed the previous record which was set in 1979 (Walter, 2020). In a survey, 2/3 of Jewish Americans felt they were "less safe today than a decade" ago (Astor, 2018). The anxiety that these people face is not unjustified. They are going through an era where they are forced to fear worshipping because of the various hate groups that are pinned against them. The pandemic has not seen a wavering in anti-Semitic behavior. In April, a man attempted to set off a bomb at a "Jewish-assisted living center" in Longmeadow, Massachusetts (Lazarus, 2019). This prompted one rabbi in the state to prompt congregants to "bring guns to the Shaloh House synagogue" (Lazarus, 2019). They fear for their safety and are being wrongfully attacked for their ethnicity and religion. The situation does not differ much in Canada either. In fact, it worsens up north. For the past few years, Jews have been the most targeted minority group within the country. While the cases have seen a downward trend, the number of cases range in the mid 300s (Walter, 2020). The two countries set of data suggest an anti-Jewish sentiment which resides in North America.

As recent as July 31st, 2020 a Jewish man in Brooklyn was attacked and struck in the face with a hard object (Lazarus, 2019). The victim was wearing a yarmulke, indicating his religion in a more direct fashion

(Lazarus, 2019). But the history of hate crimes against Jewish people in the modern age goes back even earlier. Various antisemitic organizations trace their lineage to the 18th and 19th centuries. These include the Ku Klux Klan as well as the American Nazi Party. These organizations blame Jews for ideas such as economic hardship as well as destroying the morals of society. These have led to actions such as lynchings of Jews, the drawings of swastikas on synagogues, as well as the denial of the holocaust in order to make the struggle of Jewish people appear to be less severe than it is (Lazarus, 2019).

Muslim Minorities

Islam is not a race, but it is racialized. Those with tanner complexions, who hail from specific countries are likely the same ones who are dealing with the hate crimes that befall Muslims. This issue is a prevalent one in North America. It is easy to remember the Quebec City mosque massacre which happened in just 2017 (Zine, 2020). The hate crime led to the murders of six men all with average jobs and average lives. Living as "fathers, sons, husbands, brothers" they had no specific criteria outside of religion which made them targeted. This example demonstrates a rise in hate crimes against Muslims in Canada. From 2012 to 2015 the rate of hate crimes against Muslims grew 253 percent (Zine, 2020). A recent survey done by Radio Canada Poll offers that 74 percent of Canadians want a "Canadian values test for Muslim immigrants" while "23 percent favour a ban on Muslim immigration" (Zine, 2020). Values such as this display a xenophobic tendency in the Canadian ethos which values ideas such as white supremacy by placing specific groups in duress to subvert power in place of a hierarchy.

Xenophobic attitudes towards Muslims, are just recently reaching the limelight. Following, 9-11, fears of Muslims have become a mainstream staple in North America and Europe. In Canada for example, there was a "proposed niqab ban at citizenship ceremonies" as well as a "Zero Tolerance for Barbaric Cultural Practices Act" (Zine, 2020). Both policies were aimed specifically at Muslim immigrants within Canada and while the former has gone away, the second remains but with a slight name change (Zine, 2020). It demonstrates a rise in systemic racism which requires policy change and a cultural shift to alter.

Conclusion

The common features of each hate crime presented in this article demonstrate the lack of justification used by perpetrators when attacking specific ethnic groups. In each case, the reasons behind the hate crimes were always based on speculation. More than that, the element that was most prevalent was a consistent hatred of the group itself. There was no individual in each ethnic group. They all were boxed into a label which the offender deemed appropriate. Then based on that assumed label they were then attacked. They typically never use legal methods to make their claims. However, in some of the later cases discussed legal precedence was evident within the law itself. Moreover, in most of the cases, law enforcement was used unjustifiably to physically beat down on people. So, what can we learn from these incidences? The obvious fact is that we need a change. But on a more personal level, we need to confront our biases so that they do not permeate into more obvious aspects of our lives.

Chapter 4: Historical Cases of Racialized Disease

Race and racism are a reality that so many of us grow up learning to just deal with. But if we ever hope to move past it, it can't just be on people of color to deal with it. It's up to all of us – Black, white, everyone. No matter how well-meaning we think we might be, to do the honest, uncomfortable work of rooting it out.

Michelle Obama

Race to Racism

Race has occasionally been used more-or-less as a synonym for a word that refers in some historical sense to physical, cultural, or ethnic differences among people. However, the term "race" has done far more maltreatment than aid.

Culture is defined as the learned and shared beliefs, values, and ways of life as designated in a group that is commonly transmitted to intergeneration and influences someone's way of thinking and action. Though culture is a valid descriptive variable for race differences in health conclusions, researchers must recognize that knowing one's ethnic identity does not dependably foresee principles and attitudes. Relatively, it is further significant to stipulate the cultural qualities that are being tested and include proper procedures that capture such cultural traits.

Racialization is a procedure by which societies concept races as physically unique and unequal in traditions that matter to economic, political, and social life. It comprises, choosing some individual features as expressive as meaningful signs of racial difference; categorizing individuals into races on the origin of distinctions in these characteristics; ascribing personality traits, manners and social characteristics to people grouped as members of specific races; and performing as if race designates socially substantial differences among people.

Racism can be variously defined to prejudice, discrimination, and institutions (including law), based on beliefs, physical characteristics, and cultural features and identities. Distinguishing groups of people into individuals that are superior and inferior, grouping individuals, and doing so in ways that detect the differences to be vital and biological. Racism is threatening to some racially defined groups. Such threats have frequently been construed in ways that are genocidal. Instead, race should be used as a part of social history and not the primary description.

A War on Disease or a War of Words

Ian Mackay, a virologist from the University of Queensland, confirmed that each time we get a pandemic, we are seeing something alike with previous pandemics that's reasonable enough to make judgement.

Racialized disease has been experienced for years. In the 1990s, concerns about racial unfairness and labeling appeared with growing incidence in the medical works (Geiger, 1996, 1997; King, 1996; Smith, 1998; Williams and Rucker, 2000) then initiated to be presented as matters of social justice (McGary, 1999). One of the occurrences is Swine flu disease or the H1N1 virus, which targeted Mexicans who first had the virus. Amy Fairchild, chair of sociomedical sciences at Columbia University's Mailman School of Public Health in New York City stated that it is a pattern we see frequently. It's the other race not seen as part of the state, the one who threatens it in some way that gets blamed for the disease.

The fresh discrimination and obvious racism described by Myrdal nearly six periods ago of downgrading African Americans and other minority patients to all-black hospitals, charity divisions, or the basement wards of white hospitals have extinct, but the marks of those past experiences continue, and delicate forms of differential treatment have developed (Myrdal, 1944).

The American Indian Holocaust and Survival

According to a professor of ethnic studies at the University of Colorado, Ward Churchill, the decline of the North American Indian population from an assessed of 12 million in 1,500 to hardly, 237,000 in 1,900 signifies a massive genocide, the most constant on record." On the edge of the 19th century, David E. Stannard, a historian at the University of Hawaii, wrote that local Americans had endured the ruthless human holocaust the world would have ever witnessed, thriving across two continents continuous for four centuries and devouring the lives of myriad millions of people. Additionally, on the judgment of Lenore A. Stiffarm and Phil Lane, Jr., there can be no more immense illustration of continued genocide. Undoubtedly none relating to a race of people as extensive and compound as this anywhere in the records of human history.

The sweeping control of genocide against the Indians became particularly widespread throughout the Vietnam war when historians opposed to that war began drawing equivalents among our actions in Southeast Asia and previous cases of an apparently deep-rooted American ferociousness toward non-white societies. Historian Richard Drinnon refers to the crowds under the rule of the Indian scout Kit Carson, termed them "forerunners of the Burning Fifth Marines" who placed fire to Vietnamese towns, whereas in The American Indian: The First Victim (1972), Jay David advised current readers to reminiscence how America's civilization had created "theft and murder" and "efforts toward genocide."

Typhoid Fever during Holocaust World War II

A systematic annihilation involving extensive loss of life particularly through fire. Holocaust is a Greek word, which means "sacrifice to fire", but its core definition is mass slaughter of people, especially "genocide". The Nazis believed Jews to be the lower race that posed a lethal threat to the German Volk. During the regime of Nazi on world war II, a mass assassination of loads of Jewish individuals, queer people, persons with disabilities, and other persecuted occurred. Jews were maltreated by the Nazi command early in 1933 after Adolf Hitler came to authority in Germany. During the era of the Holocaust, it is believed that Germans were "racially superior" and that the Jews considered inferior, were an unfamiliar risk to the supposed German racial community. Jewish communities were omitted from public life on September 15th, 1935 once the Nuremberg Laws were issued. These laws also denied German Jews of their citizenship and their right to marry German citizen. The Nazi government commanded all Jewish folks to dress a yellow Star of David on their clothing. This tactic secluded Jews from economic, social, cultural life and the rest of society to pressure them to emigrate and made it easier for them to be recognized and targeted (1939). Around 6 million Jewish individuals died in the Holocaust. Furthermore, millions of other individuals were also slaughtered during the Holocaust, including Roma, Jehovah's Witnesses, queer people, and individuals with disabilities.

One of the tough challenges in the sites was surviving typhoid fever and survivors formed plans to conquer the numerous challenges related to containing the disease. Both testimonies of Roman Zieglar and Leon Sniatowski shows the severe impact of the typhoid fever during the Holocaust. One of the camps Zieglar stayed in, 2,000 out of 3000 prisoners died from the occurring disease. He spent 2 weeks in a coma when he got the disease. While Leon Sniatowski had a fever that peaked at 100 degrees Fahrenheit for 2 days. This Typhoid fever grows into an epidemic in the Holocaust as the camps regularly were overloaded and there were restricted efforts to stop the virus. While considering that this is not a fatal disease, it became deadly in the Holocaust time. Nazis prioritized those who could work while with the illness. The typhus severely hampered an individual's ability to do rigorous labor. Nazis could not see any value in keeping a sick person alive if they could not work.

In 1941, as the season turned cold, the typhus broke out in the unheated residences of the beaten Jewish ghetto. This added the tedious terror to the other fears of annihilation. Numerous people were squeezed into each ghetto apartment. There was a limited possibility to bath or wash their clothes. Everyone was starving, no wonder Fleck wrote that typhus should rapidly spread in that situation. He estimated 70 percent of ghetto residents to be infected with the virus.

German public health officials first tried to fight the disease by demanding Jews to agree to delouse baths and quarantine, meaning they have to stand naked in the freezing cold, while the apartment was searched and handling over precious sets of clothes that are likely to be damaged by powerful substances.

Even in the times of widespread disease, humanity and equality vanished in this era. Power and conquering what is inferior are important during that era, that many lost mortalities.

SARS and the Media

With a single sneeze, a man attending a family wedding, infected seven other guests then took the virus to Canada, Singapore, Vietnam, and Hong Kong, as the epicenter of the virus. He was checked in to Guangdong Metropol Hotel, room 911 as preparation for the wedding.

Severe acute respiratory syndrome was confirmed to be an epidemic in Foshan, the municipality of China's Guangdong province in November 2002. Primarily, the Chinese government chooses to be silent and fails to publicize the widespread. The lack of attention and information allowed SARS to grow and spread unconstrained through the food supply. SARS was restricted within China until March 2003, after a large number of infected healthcare employees created the perfect storm for proliferation.

In 2003, the spread of local news about the SARS outbreak had led to a racial panic in the community and had serious health consequences, with over 8,000 infected by respiratory disease and 816 deaths. The Southeast Asian communities in Canada faced serious social and economic implications. Residents of Toronto enacted an informal boycott to the Chinese community which stigmatized and discriminated against Asian Canadians. Anti-Asian racism, blown by the mainstream media, led to major financial losses for many Asian-owned small businesses with losses up to eighty percent of their income, and CBC News reported businesses in Toronto's Chinatown reported their customers dropping by 70 to 90 percent from the SARS scare. Additionally, the Ontario government's post-SARS commission found cases of Asian or Chinese workers getting terminated from their jobs and Chinese tenants unlawfully kicked out by their landlords. There were also regular events of verbal and physical violence against individuals assumed to be Chinese.

There was a reported occurrence in New Jersey during the SARS epidemic. Artists with Chinese backgrounds were denied access to a middle school. This suggests that SARS becomes part of a national lexicon, fear, rumor, suspicion, and misinformation can threaten racial harmony in any country (Newman and Zhao, 2003).

The Chinese people were viewed as the perpetrators for starting the spread of this infectious disease. As the media played its one final important role in connecting the incidence of the virus to the Asian people. Several articles of Canadian published the name of the first diagnosed patient with SARS. They even reported the names of the family members. They coined the patient as the "super spreader" who carried SARS from Hong Kong to Canada and was believed to be responsible for exposing the disease for as many as 155 residents. One of those noticeable visual references to the SARS outbreak was the face mask worn by an Asian. Images of the Asian wearing face mask marked the Chinese, Southeast, and East Asian groups for discrimination and alienation.

An extensive variety of articles were published from March 31 to April 21, 2003, containing a plethora of large published images of Chinese citizens in Hong Kong wearing medical masks while conducting their daily routines. Photos were accompanied by labels threatening the spread of SARS, such as "Will SARS Strike Here?" and "Settlers Quarantined to Contain Disease." Each of these articles was issued in Canada, images correspondingly portrayed white clinical masks adorned by Chinese women in Hong Kong while walking down the street and, Chinese children showing academic lessons in a classroom. These cover page spreads were exaggerating and misleading. By displaying images of Asians put on the white masks, the media has lured the general public to associate the disease to Asians. Associated with SARS as a mysterious "Oriental" entity, Asian publics were assumed to be plagued and posed a serious health risk to society.

Chapter 5: COVID-19 Context and Hate Crimes against Asians

During this global pandemic caused by the virus recognized as COVID-19, we continue to fight against another disease, one that has been with us since the nation's founding: "white supremacy". What equivalent efforts have been made to prevent the spread of toxicity of racism across the country? Through the emergence of COVID-19, the mounting anti-Asian violence has pushed many Asians out of their own communities to take an eye at the nature of white supremacy and our involvement in it. It is not new to the Asian people to be hated with this emerged disease that had arisen. The blame will constantly be where the virus originated, and since the SARS era, Asians were the ones to be accountable of the disease's spreading and confining. In eight weeks since COVID-19's inception, thousands of individuals have reported hate incidents to Asians ranging from verbal harassment to physical assaults. What Asian communities have realized, especially those who believed they were protected by educational privilege and economic capital – is that they are not exempt from racism. There were several reported cases of hate crimes throughout this pandemic.

Shown below are some reported cases from February 2020 until June 2020.

Timeline of reported cases relating to anti-Asian Hate Crime

Date	Location	Cases	Source
2-Feb	New York, NY	One witness stated to a report that she heard a man calling the woman a "diseased b****", the Asian woman was attacked in the subway station for wearing a mask.	CNN
12-Feb	Plymouth, IN	Kao Lor and Lee Lor, were traveling through Indiana and tried to get a room at a Super 8 Motel. The Super 8 employee questioned Lor if he was Chinese. When Lor asked why he was required to identify, the employee responded, "Because of the coronavirus going around. And anyone from China, I am told, has to be picked up and quarantined for two weeks."	WBND
13-Feb	Los Angeles, CA	In the San Fernando Valley, a 16-year-old student, who is of Asian descent, was physically assaulted by classmates due to coronavirus fears	CBS-Los Angeles
22-Feb	San Francisco, CA	An old Asian man was physically attacked while gathering recyclables close to a housing project. The event was recorded and shared widely on social media. In the video, one person can be heard declaring, "I hate Asians." Dwayne Grayson was detained on suspicion of robbery, elder abuse and committing a hate crime, as well as a trial violation for a previous robbery.	San Francisco Chronicle
27-Feb	Philadelphia, PA	A young man and woman were physically assaulted by a group of teenagers at a SEPTA station in what seems to be a racially driven anti-Asian attack.	NextShark

1-Mar	New York, NY	An Asian man was standing on the road smoking a cigarette when somebody threw a container of liquid on him, resulting in a physical fight.	NextShark
4-Mar	Brooklyn, NY	Video shows a man on the subway arguing with a fellow passenger, who is Asian, and then spraying Febreze air freshener on the Asian passenger.	ABC-NY
6-Mar	Garden City, CA	Two students at Bolsa Grande High School videoed themselves verbally harassing and mocking Vietnamese American classmates, yelling "coronavirus" at them during an International Week assembly	OC Register
6-Mar	Cumberland County, PA	A passerby on campus harassed and hurled racist insults at an Asian-American student at a local college	Reported to ADL
7-Mar	New York, NY	A 13-year-old boy spat at a 59-year-old Asian man and allegedly saying Chinese people have COVID-19. The same boy attacked the same man again on March 10 in a similar incident	CBS-NY

9-Mar	San Francisco, CA	A woman told the correspondents that while walking to the fitness center she was harassed by a man who yelled curses about China and encouraged a passing bus to "run them over." The man then spat at her.	New York Times
10-Mar	New York, NY	A student from Korea was attacked while entering a building on West 34th Street. The suspect asked her, "Where's your (swearword) mask?" She then proceeded to grip the victim by the hair and punch her in the face. The lady allegedly also told the victim, "You've got coronavirus, you Asian (expletive)." NYPD is inspecting the assault as a probable bias crime.	ABC-NY
10-Mar	New York, NY	NYPD arrested a 13-year-old boy and charged him with assault and serious harassment as hate crimes after he approached a 59-year-old Asian man from behind and made anti-Asian statements. The assaulter allegedly told the victim to go back to his country and remark on coronavirus. He also kicked the victim	CBS-NY
10-Mar	Charlottesville VA	The Mainland Student Network at the University of Virginia reported that two Chinese international undergraduates were attacked by assaulter (s) who threw raw eggs at them from a moving automobile	Facebook
12-Mar	Milwaukee, WI	Komeng Yang recounted in a Facebook post that some passengers in the bus avoided him and kept their distance "because of the fear of the virus." After he sneezed caused by a pollen from a passenger's flowers, someone allegedly said, "Kick him off the bus."	Facebook

13-Mar	Miami, FL	Video shows an elderly Asian woman being chased with a bottle of Purell and a man yelling, "Come here! You need some hand sanitizer. Sanitize your ass!"	NextShark
14-Mar	Midland, TX	A Burmese man and his two children, ages six and two, were attacked and stabbed at a Sam's Club by a 19-year-old man. The alleged assailant admitted to targeting the family because he believed the family was Chinese and infecting people with coronavirus. The assailant was charged with three counts of attempted capital murder and one count aggravated assault.	The Daily Beast
16-Mar	New York, NY	An Asian woman was physically assaulted by a woman who accused her of spreading the coronavirus. The alleged perpetrator was arrested and charged with a hate crime	New York Post
21-Mar	Naperville, IL	A Chinese American man was jogging when he was confronted by two women who accused him of having the virus and told him to "go back to China." They also threw a log and spat on him.	WBEZ Chicago
23-Mar	Des Moines, IA	An Asian American woman was waiting in line at a bakery when a white couple said, "Oh gosh, not here" and "fled" to a different line after they saw she was Asian.	Des Moines Register

24-Mar	San Francisco, CA	A man yelled at a Filipino-American man, using an anti-Asian derogatory term.	Twitter
25-Mar	Woodbury, MN	A woman returned home to find this flier posted on her door: "We're watching you fucking chinks take the Chinese virus back to China. We don't want you here infecting us with your diseases!!!!!!!"	Facebook
25-Mar	South Bend, IN	A student at the University of Notre Dame posted racist, anti-Asian, anti-Chinese comments on their Facebook page. The student also wrote "Go home" on the Facebook page of an international student from China.	The Observer
26-Mar	Seattle, WA	A Chinese restaurant in the Chinatown-International District of Seattle was vandalized	NBC News
27-Mar	Evanston, IL	A spray-paint with words "Make China Pay" was found inside a bus shelter.	Reported to ADL

27-Mar	Cerritos, CA	A Korean American woman was insulted in the parking lot of Walmart by a man who called her a "bitch asshole" and threatened to hit her.	Reported to ADL
27-Mar	Martinsville, IN	A man of Korean background was denied entry into a gas station and told to "never come back." The gas station attendants reportedly stated to the police that "anyone of Chinese origin was not permitted in the store."	WISH-TV
27-Mar	San Angelo, TX	A Korean student at Angelo State University returned to his dormitory room to discover that someone had placed posters about COVID-19 on his door.	San Angelo Live
28-Mar	New York, NY	An Asian woman walking her dogs was verbally bullied by two publics who called her "the virus."	NextShark
28-Mar	Evanston, IL	"Chinese virus" was located spray-painted on a jetty on the Northwestern University campus	Reported to ADL

29-Mar	Bronx, NY	Three teenage girls harassed and used an umbrella to assault an Asian woman, saying, "You caused coronavirus, bitch."	New York Post
3-Apr	Seymour, CT	A Chinese food restaurant received racist and threatening phone calls from callers who blamed the owners, who are Chinese, for the COVID-19 pandemic. The callers also threatened to shoot the owners	Valley New Haven Independent
4-Apr	Edison, NJ	A group of juveniles encircled an Asian woman and criticized her with racial slurs before hitting her in the back of the head.	NJ Advance Media
17-Apr	Albuquerque, NM	A Chinese American reported that while at a supermarket another shopper singled him out and asked him to "stay away."	Reported to ADL
18-Apr	Atlanta, GA	A logo of Winnie the Pooh using chopsticks to dine a bat and the terms "Wuhan Plague" was found outside of a coffee shop. The plaque was also allegedly displayed at other places around East Atlanta on April 13 and April 16.	The Atlanta Journal-Constitution

25-Apr	Chesapeake, VA	A Chinese restaurant owner was harassed by an individual who threw water on her and her husband. The owner of the restaurant also reported that someone painted "Go back to China" on her car.	The Virginian-Pilot
26-Apr	Queens, NY	An Asian woman in Rego Park was harassed by a man who yelled curses and told her, "You're the one who brought the virus here." After the woman attempted to make a recording of him on her cellphone, he grabbed her phone away.	Patch
1-May	Hoboken, NJ	A spray-painted anti-Asian graffiti was reported on the sidewalk outside an apartment building.	Patch
3-May	New York, NY	An Asian man was harassed on the subway by a stranger who shouted at him, "You're infected China boy, you need to get off the train." The assaulter then grasped the victim and attempted to pull him out of his seat.	NY Daily News
3-May	Pasadena, CA	A man was arrested by a police officer who pitched a beverage while yelling racial slurs at several Asian American individuals.	Pasadena Now

5-May	St. Louis, MO	Displayed in a restaurant is a pinata shaped of coronavirus with a racist depiction of an Asian on it.	Riverfront Times
12-May	Stevens Point, WI	A man was detained after using racial slurs against Asian shoppers in a grocery store. According to police "the purchasers were called names and bullied for wearing masks because of their race."	WSAW
15-May	New York, NY	An Asian woman was verbally harassed by fellow subway passengers for not wearing her mask "properly." The passenger yelled at the victim, "You fucking Chinese don't speak English! Go back to China!" She also slapped the victim's phone away.	NY Daily News
13-Jun	Queens, NY	At a Bayside 7-Eleven, a man made an anti-Asian remarks regarding the COVID-19 pandemic and then verbally harassed an Asian customer whom he also allegedly pushed.	NY Daily News

The virus does not choose age, gender, or race. Anyone can get infected, so it is on people's responsibility to prevent being diseased. We cannot avoid having some sort of virus, but we can prevent it from spreading.

Most people take advantage of other's weaknesses instead of helping to support them. We cannot see the unity of each other, different races holding on each other's hands. Values are conveyed from generations to generations. If racism prevails, there will be no equality visible in the countries disregarding it. Some other reported cases including New York, California, and Texas, East Asians have been spat on, punched, kicked, or worst being stabbed. In California, a senior was struck with an iron bar, and a teenager was taken to hospital after being physically assaulted.

Whether they have been confronted with total violence, bullying or more sinister forms of social or political abuse, a spike in anti-Asian prejudice has left many Asians wondering whether they fit in "American society". A3PCON Community asks the government's protection for the Asian community to avoid such anti-Asian hate crime. We are all part of this world, and part of God's big family. Each family member differs from each other, but they still help and love each other.

Chapter 6: Increasing Prevalence of Hate Crimes Against Asians

Some incidents reached the bar of hate crimes. Authorities in New York City and Los Angeles declare that hate incidents against people of Asian background have escalated, while a reporting Centre run by advocacy groups and San Francisco State University says it collected over 1,700 statements of coronavirus-related discrimination from at least 45 US states since it began in March. Report reviews 673 reports of coronavirus discrimination give in to on the CAA/A3PCON "Stop AAPI Hate" website from March 19-25, 2020. Even without much exposure, A3PCON have already received a solid answer from the community, who want their voices to be heard.

Emerging trends include:
• Nearly 100 reports daily, with 5.5% from limited-English speakers
• Women are three times more likely to report harassment than men
• Asian Americans of different ethnicities are racially profiled; 61% of the reports are from non-Chinese
• Verbal harassment and name calling are the most frequently reported type of discrimination,
making up over 2/3 of reports
• With shelter-in-place policies, Asian Americans are more likely to face coronavirus discrimination in businesses, especially stores, rather than at schools and public transit as previously observed

Examples of the types of discrimination are found after the tables which are data collected based on surveys.

Type of discrimination %	
Barred from Establishment	2.40%
Barred from Transportation	1.00%
Coughed/Spat Upon	2.70%
Online	2.20%
Physical Assault	10.00%
Shunning	23.50%
Verbal Harassment	67.30%
Workplace Discrimination	4.60%
Other	7.40%

Reason for Discrimination %	
Ethnicity	65.50%
Face Mask	14.10%
Food	4.80%
Gender	6.40%
Language	6.40%
Race	89.50%

Religion	1.20%

Site of Discrimination %	
Business	47.00%
Online	8.90%
Private Residence	7.00%
Public Park	15.50%
Public Street	0.60%
Public Transit	15.20%
School	4.20%
University	1.90%
Other	1.20%

Language of Respondent %	
Japanese	1.50%
Korean	0.90%
Chinese Traditional	1.20%
Chinese Simplified	1.90%

English	94.50%

Age %	
10s	5.30%
20s	30.30%
30s	32.20%
40s	17.90%
50s	7.90%
60s	6.00%
70s	0.50%

Gender %	
Women	73.60%
Men	25.70%
Non - binary	0.60%

Ethnicity %	
African American	0.30%

Asian	12.80%
Burmese	0.10%
Cambodian	0.70%
Chinese	38.60%
Filipino	4.20%
Hmong	4.60%
Indonesian	0%
Iu Mien	0.30%
Japanese	5.30%
Korean	16.50%
Lao	1.30%
Multiracial	0.90%
Mongolian	0.30%
Taiwanese	5.50%
Thai	0.70%
Vietnamese	7%
White	4.50%
Other	0.70%

Some reported statements of harassed Asian individuals

1. Barred from Establishment

• An Asian was shouted and harassed by the cashier, workers, as well as customers at the store to get out of the store. "You Chinese bring the virus here and you dare ask people to keep social distance guidelines."

• "I was not seen by the employee at my local post office where I have been a regular customer for over 20 years. After patiently waiting as she pointed to others behind me for nearly 45 minutes, I approached the desk when she prompted me to take several steps backwards in a very hostile tone. She had not requested any of the prior customers that had gone ahead of me, and they were also all non-Asians. The sting of her racism and coldness towards me made me feel less than and frankly, dehumanized."

2. Barred from Transportation

• Called for Lyft XL from Int'l Terminal Pickup. Lyft driver arrives. Rolls down window. Mumbles something and speeds off, refusing to give me a ride. It was snowing and I was with my 18-month-old son and partner returning from Costa Rica.

• 2 separate Uber drivers would not pick me up due to my race. Each time, the driver would arrive, look at me, and speed off quickly to cancel the ride a minute later. The second driver had a face mask on, and he slowed down enough to look at me and shake his head and wave a hand at me rejecting the ride.

3. Coughed/Spat Upon

• "I took a walk with a friend of mine in Visalia, CA. While we were passing a group of 4 men, one of them coughed into me, not once, but TWICE, without covering his mouth. As I turned my head back, they all burst out laughing. They then backed away.

• "Walking to work, older black man walking towards my direction yelled fucking Chinese disease and suddenly stepped near me and spat at me hitting my coat, scarf and face. A lot of disgusting saliva. The police nearby when I told him he said I could go after the aggressor who was still in plain sight. A younger black man who saw everything backed me up. The policemen were useless.

4. Online

• I posted on my timeline "Mexican wall, Chinese virus, what's next
40

America" and people started commenting about how the Chinese are to blame because it started from China. The post was highly destructive, and it made me feel uncomfortable, so I decided to delete it.

• I was engaged in an online discussion about the source of COVID19 and got hanged up on by a group of 3 men and one woman. At the end, the woman accused me of being patient 0 and a virus transmitter

5. Physical Assault

• A white male assaulted me by throwing his drink in my face and shouting things like "they should be banned" and "they're all disgusting." I then saw him a couple hours later; this time inside the building, rather than outside on the sidewalk, walking around the store. I filed a police report the following day with the Police Station

• I was walking home and someone in a pickup truck threw a bottle at me really hard. He missed.

6. Shunning

• I walked into the train carriage and immediately two teenage girls started screaming and "eewing" and making a show of covering their mouths and faces with a scarf then stood up and ran to the other end of the carriage (which was more crowded) jeering at me.

• As I was walking to my bus, a white, middle-aged man screamed at me to "wear a

respirator" because I'm Asian. And when I was on the bus, a middle-aged woman sitting across from me kept gazing at me while holding a rosary in front of her. After a few minutes of this, she moved a few seats away from me while keeping eye contact with me.

7. Verbal Harassment/Name Calling

• Young "white" girl told her parents she was going to "Die" (repeatedly) and her parents

asked why? And she said of Coronavirus and pointed in my direction.

• When I was walking in the subway station, a black guy said "F*****

Asian" to me unexpectedly.

8. Workplace Discrimination

• I'm reporting for a family. My brother in law was asked to go home because someone at his work said his wife had Covid-19. He was not asked if this was true before dismissing him for the day. His wife does not have Covid-19. Both him and his wife are Asian

American.

• In office team meeting, I found myself being a target of snarky comments about being linked to the cause and the spread of the coronavirus. I'm not Chinese and I haven't traveled internationally in years. It was ignorance at its best and comments were taken as good humor by others in the room.

Chapter 7: Racist Language Around COVID-19

How can Asian-American or Asians that are not in their hometown or country spread the virus, even if they did not even go back to their native country during the pandemic? Is it already part of our nature to look at whom we blame for anything that happens, even if they weren't really the one to be blamed for?

Prejudice is a great time saver. You can form opinions without having to get the facts.

E.B White

• Early February – Pasadena, CA: Tzi Ma, a Chinese American actor claimed that a man yelled at him that he should be quarantined. (Source: Good Morning America

• February 1 - Los Angeles, CA: An Asian woman was exposed to an anti-Asian racist rage about coronavirus from another commuter as taking the Metro. The man uttered "Every disease has ever come from China, homie. Everything comes from China because they're fucking disgusting." (Source: Twitter)

• February 5 - Los Angeles, CA: An eighth-grade Asian-American at Walter Reed Middle School was directed to the nurse's office after he unexpectedly cough from choking on water. Afterwards, the nurse brought him back to class. The other pupils teased him that he had coronavirus. (Source: FOX-Los Angeles)

• Early March – Los Angeles, CA: A woman testified that a man tailed her while she was jogging, and shouted that because she is Chinese, she was at fault for transporting the disease to the United States. (Source:

Los Angeles Times)

• Early March – Orange County, CA: It was knowledgeable in an op-ed that first of March, an Asian-American fourth grade student's classmates criticized him for suffering from coronavirus. (Source: Los Angeles Times)

• March 7 - Syracuse, NY, Syracuse University: An advertisement with material about preventing the increase of the coronavirus was vandalized with racist words directed to Chinese individuals. (Source: The Daily Orange)

• March 9 - Fresno, CA: An Asian man's vehicle was vandalized "F***, Asians and Coronavirus ." (Source: ABC 30)

• March 10 - New York, NY: Ed Park wrote in The New Yorker magazine that a young black man told him to get the f*** away from him. Park asked the man if he was referring to him and the man responded: "Yes, you, fucking Chinese motherfucker, don't fucking get me sick." (Source: The New Yorker)

• March 11 - Seattle, WA: A student at the University of Washington told reporters that he had been troubled the earlier week while commuting on the light rail to university. According to Kim, another passenger yelled at him about Chinese carrying diseases to the United States. (Source: Crosscut)

• March 11 - Washington DC: A Cambodian-American man was at a 7-Eleven when a fellow shopper named him a "chink". (Source: NextShark)

• March 12 – New York, NY: An Asian man was in a restroom at Penn Station when he was verbally harassed by a man who called him a "Chinese fuck" and said, "I hope you die by the coronavirus." The perpetrator also spat on the victim. (Source: Patch)

• March 12 - Queens, NY: Police arrested Raoul Ramos and charged him with aggravated harassment as a hate crime after he allegedly harassed and pushed a 47-year-old Asian man who was walking with his 10-year-old son in the Forest Hills area. Ramos approached the pair and started screaming, "Where the [expletive] is your mask?" He also referred to them as "You f****** Chinese." (Source: New York Post)

• March 12 - Albuquerque, NM: (Date approximate) At the University of New Mexico, an international student from China returned to his dorm room in Lobo Village to discover plastic covering his door and a sign that read, "Caution, Keep Out, Quarantine." (Albuquerque, NM). Source: KOB 4

• March 12 - Albuquerque, NM: (Date approximate) Kay Bounkeua, Executive Director of NM Asian Family Center, told local news that while walking into her office someone on the street yelled at her to go back to where she came from. (Sour March 13 – Pasadena, CA: A movie poster for Mulan was defaced with graffiti that showed a mask over the titular character's face and the message "Toxic made in Wuhan." (Source: NBC News)

• March 13 – Pasadena, CA: A movie poster for Mulan was defaced with graffiti that depicted a mask over the supposed character's face and the message "Toxic made in Wuhan." (Source: NBC News)

• March 15 – Los Angeles, CA: A Filipino-American woman was harassed by a woman on the street who exclaimed, "Please don't give me the virus" (Source: Twitter)

• March 15 – New York, NY: A man approached an Asian woman on the subway and asked, "You're Chinese, why did you bring Corona to America?" (Source: Facebook)

• March 15 – Louisville, CO: Union Jack Liquor changed the note on their shelter to read "Firestone $14.88 Thanks China." "14/88" associations two popular white supremacist numeric hate symbols. (Source: Colorado Hometown Weekly)

• March 15 – Davie, FL: An Asian woman who works as an instrumentalist had harassing and racist text messages telling her that she would not be hired any longer until she gave in her "Chinese passport and renounced your Chinese citizenship." (Source: NextShark)

• March 16 – Fresno, CA: An Asian American woman was harassed while buying diapers. She was told to move out of the way and then denoted to exercising a racial slur. (Source: The Fresno Bee)

• March 16 – Daly City, CA: An Asian man coughed while shopping at Target and was verbally harassed by other purchasers. (Source: NextShark)

• March 16 – Vestal, NY: A student at Binghamton University revealed that someone had submitted a racist response to a public Google form she had posted for an occasion. The submission included anti-Asian terms and referred to the coronavirus. (Source: Pipe Dream)

• March 17 – New York, NY: Jiayang Fan, a staff journalist at The New Yorker magazine, reported being vocally harassed outside her apartment by a passerby who continually yelled "Fucking Chinese" at her, and called her a "Chinese bitch." (Source: Twitter)

• March 17 – Albuquerque, NM: A local Asian restaurant was vandalized with a spray-painted message that read "Trucha with the coronavirus." "Trucha" is slang in Spanish for "beware" or "watch out."(Source: KOB 4)

• March 19 – Brooklyn, NY: Oswald Jones, 60, targeted a 26-year-old Asian woman, allegedly yelling "Go back to China" and "You are dirty, get your temperature checked," before attempting to punch her and steal her cellphone. Source: (NY Daily News)

• March 20 – Los Angeles, CA: CNN journalist Kyung Lah was preparing for a broadcast when a man approached her and used a racial slur. (Source: CNN)

• March 21 – Huntington Beach, CA: A flier that read, "You guys are Chinese Viruses" and "Get out of our country" was posted on a family's front door and left on their car. (Source: Reported to ADL)

• March 24 – Brooklyn, NY: In a subway station, someone spat on an Asian man and yelled, "You fucking Chinese, spreading the coronavirus. You people got the virus." Source: NY Daily News)

• March 24 – Columbia, MD: An Asian-American family was walking on a neighborhood trail when they were verbally harassed by neighbors who shouted at them, "Coronavirus, coronavirus! Asian pig!" (Source: Baltimore Sun)

• March 24 – Madison, WI: Anti-Chinese messages referring to COVID-19 as the "Chinese Virus" were found written in chalk on the University of Wisconsin-Madison campus. (Source: Milwaukee Journal Sentinel)

• March 24 – San Francisco, CA: A man yelled at a Filipino-American man, using an anti-Asian derogatory term. (Source: Twitter)

• March 25 – South Bend, IN: A student at the University of Notre Dame posted racist, anti-Asian, anti-Chinese comments on their Facebook page. The student also wrote "Go home" on the Facebook page of an international student from China. (Source: The Observer)

• March 27 – Evanston, IL: Someone spray-painted the words "Make China Pay" inside a bus shelter. (Source: Reported to ADL)

• March 27 – Asheville, NC: A cooking class held on Zoom by an Asian American chef was disrupted by an unknown person who yelled anti-Asian and homophobic epithets. (Source: Citizen-Times)

• March 27 – Martinsville, IN: A man of Korean descent was denied entry into a gas station and told to "never come back." The gas station attendants reportedly told police that "anyone of Chinese descent was not allowed in the store." (Source: WISH-TV)

• March 28 – Evanston, IL: "Chinese virus" was discovered spray-painted on a dock on the Northwestern University campus. (Source: Reported to ADL)

• March 28 – New York, NY: An Asian woman walking her dogs was vocally bullied by two people who termed her "the virus." (Source: NextShark)

• March 30 – Yakima, WA: An Asian buffet restaurant was vandalized with graffiti that involved an ethnic insult and a note that read, "Take the corona back." (Source: YakTriNews)

• March 31 – Webster Groves, MO: American Identity Movement, an alt right group, circulated propaganda that read encouraged their group and presented a Corona beer bottle with the coronavirus germ and state: "Immigration kills," and "Made in China." (Source: ADL identified)

• March 31 – Philadelphia, PA: Several Asian American homes obtained a letter that referenced eating bats and pangolin and encouraged the recipients to burn themselves alive. Source: WHYY

• April 1 – Pittsburgh, PA: (Date approximate) An Asian American woman was at a grocery store when she was ordered by another shopper to shop with her own kind and that she should be rounded up with the virus and shipped back to China.(Source: Pittsburgh's Action News 4)

• April 2 – Cherry Hill, NJ: A Vietnamese American man was walking his dog when he was orally harassed by a stranger who yelled that he caused the coronavirus and needed to get the fuck out of there. Source: WHYY

• April 5 – San Marcos, CA: An Asian woman was verbally harassed in a Costco parking lot by an anonymous male who blamed the woman and Chinese citizens for the virus. (Source: FOX 16)

• April 7 – Amherst, MA: (Date approximate) In a note to the Amherst College community, the president of the college reported that two Asian students at Amherst College had apparently been the targets of verbal harassment in the town of Amherst. (Source: Amherst College)

• April 8 – Houston, TX: A woman verbally harassed some employees of a Vietnamese restaurant, telling them to get out of their country. (Source: ABC-13)

• April 10 – New York, NY: A Korean restaurant was defaced with graffiti that state, "Stop eating dogs." (Source: NY Eater)

• April 10 – New York, NY: A Zoom session held by an Asian American organization was disturbed by unknown individuals who wrote racist and anti-Asian slurs in the chat function. (Source: Reported to ADL)

• April 12 – Seattle, WA: Patriot Front, an alt right group, posted propaganda around Seattle's International District targeting Asian American/Pacific Islander businesses. (Source: ADL identified)

• April 15 – Newton, MA: A high school advanced placement Chinese class held on Zoom was disrupted by individuals who targeted the students and teachers using racial slurs and loud mock-Chinese, and posting "vile, hate-filled images." (Source: Boston Globe)

• April 16 – Brooklyn, NY: An Asian woman was walking on the boulevard in the Bedford-Stuyvesant neighborhood when two men harassed her with remarks about Chinese people and called her a "F*****g freak." (Source: Reported to ADL)

• April 17 – Philadelphia, PA: (Date approximate) An Asian-owned restaurant was vandalized with spray-painted graffiti that included the racial slur "Chink." Source: WHYY

• April 19 – San Francisco, CA: An Asian American lady was harassed while walking her dogs. She was advised to go back to whatever f****** country she came from and that nasty people should stay in f****g Asia. (Source: Facebook)

• April 20 – Orange County, CA: During a second-grade class held on Zoom, a pupil expressed to the class that he does not like "China or Chinese people because they started this quarantine." (Source: Facebook)

• April 22 – San Jose, CA: Five Asian-Owned businesses were vandalized in nearby neighborhoods of San Jose. (Source: East Bay Times)

• April 25 – Pasadena, CA: An Asian man was walking with a companion when a motorist drove past and yelled at them, "Fucking Asians, motherfuckers. You brought this disease here." Source: NextShark

• May 14 – San Luis Obispo, CA: The Cal Poly Chinese Student Association's Zoom conference was interrupted by an unidentified participant who drew swastikas and filled the chat box with xenophobic remarks accusing the pandemic on Chinese. (Source: KSBY)

• May 17 – Contra Costa, CA: A farm stand displayed a racist sign that read "Fresh bat soup" and "Thank you China." (Source: Reported to ADL)

• May 22 – San Leandro, CA: A woman was arrested after posting handwritten flysheets on homes that read, in part, "If you are a woman or man and was born in other country, return, go back to your land immediately, fast, with urgency" and "In this place, no Asians allowed." (Source: SF Gate)

• May 30 – San Mateo, CA: Racist anti-Chinese letters were located in the Laurelwood neighborhood, written on utility boxes and poles. (Source: The Daily Journal)

• May 23 – Seattle, WA: A man harassed an Asian at a park and an Asian woman in her car, saying, "Where are you from...where is your ID?", and "Chinese disease...they bring it here!" Later, the man allegedly yelled anti-Asian remarks inside an Asian restaurant. (Source: King 5)

• June 6 – Denver, CO: Two Asian American were verbally confronted while walking on the way by a female who stated that they "smell like shit" and "You guys are all disgusting! You all!" (Source: Reported to ADL)

• June 3 – Brooklyn, NY: Conspiratorial anti-Chinese fliers were posted in Bay Ridge. The flyers blamed the spread of COVID-19 on Chinese settlers. (Source: Gothamist)

• June 14 – Newark, DE: Fliers directing Asian and Asian American pupils were found at off-campus housing at the University of Delaware, Newark. The flyers contained the note "Kill China Virus." (Source: WDEL)

• June 17 – Wyckoff, NJ: A Chinese restaurant was vandalized with graffiti that read, "coronavirus" and "COVID-19." (Source: NorthJersey. com)

Pandemic tests everyone's humanity, patience, and how people think. Being superior to other races does not give you power, it gives you the chance to be a "role model". Without the so-called "race" exist, we all are equal human beings created on different islands. We should all have equal rights with everything on this earth. With no racism, everybody will be at peace and live in harmony without hatred. We are in a different generation, we should not let hate and inhuman activities keep on happening, the racism matter should be resolved urgently.

Chapter 8: The Racialization of Coronavirus

The COVID-19 pandemic has reinforced a recurring theme in the study of diseases, the racialization of disease. This time however, racial hierarchies were propagated differently. The COVID-19 Pandemic's racialization was not through colonialism, imperialism, or slavery. In fact, a single driver: mainstream media, holds much of the weight of the burden [1].

Racialization of Coronavirus and the media

Coronavirus is a global crisis, a pandemic that received mass media coverage. At the center of the attention, however, lies racism. From the article headings and figure captions, to the actual content of media reports, the rhetoric surrounding discussions of the pandemic, the curve, demographics, and pathophysiology of the coronavirus, all allude to race. Header images, in particular, are being consistently suggestive with East Asian individuals being the focus [2]. Also, numerous media reports went so far in presenting a narrative that demonizes a particular race, often the East Asians, that a foreign government would be assumed the focus of the press release instead of the matter at hand, the pandemic. In these releases, terms such as "communism" and "authoritarianism" would be highlighted as opposed to medical terminology. Repetition and flow, narrative arcs almost, drive forward a race focus.

Racialization of Coronavirus and Political figures

Politics greatly shape the lives each and every one of leads. Political correctness, economics, international relations, and really politically discourse, influence our actions, feelings, goals, and daily doings. Politics are presented to average citizens through politicians. Though politicians ideally should not have conflicting interests with the greater good of community, bias and corruption may and often does penetrate. The concern is that the views of political figures greatly direct the collective opinions of many matters, the COVID-19 pandemic included of course. However, many politicians look past the immense responsibility they have of using their voices and platforms for good, and poorly present ideas to the public. For example, a member of parliament (MP) may speak of the pandemic while blaming the Chinese for the public health problems escalating globally. The speech delivered by the aforementioned MP would be covered by the press, could promote further negative discussion, and even push for the general public to hold such attitudes. In this example, the MP could easily be replaced with a party leader, a publicist, journalist, or even a prime minister or president. In fact, the channel of discussion does not even need to be particularly "political." The faith and reliance the general public consciously or subconsciously hold in the drivers of political discourse, the political figures that represent us, is strong enough for even clearly pseudo-scientific ideas to "legitimize" and propel through the endorsements of politicians. The language, in particular, coined by politicians for discussing the pandemic has been widely spread amongst the media outlets, and likely, the audience or general public as well at some point. A prominent example of a politician coined reference relevant to the COVID-19 pandemic discussion, includes the "Wuhan virus." Politicians can add to the chaos and stress experienced by citizens through throwing shade at other countries and governments, escalating tensions felt between the countries, making matters complicated for international students and visitors from the specific countries, and racializing the pandemic further.

Racialization of Coronavirus and Social Media

The racialization of diseases continues to propagate through socialization. Nowadays much of the socialization that occurs is done through social media. Social media facilitates extremely fast debates, trends, and ideas in general. Hashtags, groups, memes, posts, comments, and replies can carry much information, disseminate it, and foster an association, even if merely perceived, between aspects of a disease and a race, ethnic group, or population.

Tedros Adhanom Ghebreyesus, the director-general of the World

Health Organization (WHO), recently expressed a dire need to combat what he calls the "coronavirus infodemic." The infodemic is the public discussion of the pandemic. Primarily being channeled via social media, the infodemic is a cause for misinformation transmission and public confusion. A great cause for concern in terms of this infodemic is the racist remarks circulated regarding the pandemic.

Racist content shared through social media often reiterates existing stereotypes and biases [3]. Social media can quickly ingrain rumours, conspiracy theories, and myths in the minds of consumers, making the targets or "antagonists" of the negative content prone to physical harm and cyber-bullying.

Since the sheer number of active users is so significant on these social media platforms, the audience is intercepting the information, or misinformation projected, extremely quickly, to an extent far greater than simple messaging, email, or phone calls could have allowed in other times. Anonymity further allows people to feel rather comfortable in posting unfiltered thoughts and opinions, many of which may be xenophobic and racist in nature. During these difficult times where government bodies, policymakers, and professionals overall, are expending their time and energy to attend to the physical safety and healthcare of populations, censorship is particularly difficult. With censorship being somewhat lagging, social media users have yet another layer of cushioning to carry on in racializing the pandemic, and feeling rather easy in doing so as penalties and punishments for such negativity are represented by slim odds.

It is essential to note however that social media platforms are also being used to facilitate healthy discussion. In fact, news stories are rather conveniently read online. Scientific, peer-reviewed articles and research papers are also accessible via online journals and databases. Videos published online by medical experts, scientists, and public health professionals can be watched and reviewed by anyone sitting home with access to a device with wifi. So, accurate, relatively objective, or unbias, evidence-based information is also made accessible by technology and widespread by social media. Additionally, many social media users use their voice to break down racist messages being constructed and shared on the very same platforms they are initially shared on. Many users take time out of their schedules to create infographics that debunk racist myths, clip art that highlights the repercussions of racializing, and write detailed blogs and posts to discuss how terrible the racialization of the pandemic really is.

Racialized Responses and Mental Health

The racism prevalent in the workforce and otherwise, of course has severe harmful influences to those targeted in particular [4]. Businesses, schools, and institutions have been closed, reopened, remodelled to online modes of delivery, yet the groups targeted in terms of racism may still be well subject to intense emotional damage. In fact, many of the news reports published in recent times discuss the frustration experienced by individuals in general. Those subject to an additional bombardment of misery should be kept in mind for sociological, psychological, and anthropological research conducted in the time of the pandemic. The groups subject to racism should also be an important part of the headlines surfacing in news forums. It is imperative that healthy discussion be circulating regarding mental health with people of color, the black lives matter movement, and discriminated minorities in mind. Nonetheless, in such a trying time, it is key for all individuals to have access to metal health support and for there to be a focus on research conducted to understand the mental health of individuals living through the pandemic [5].

Demographics and Socioeconomic Distribution of Disease

Even if one zooms out of the COVID-19 pandemic and analyzes diseases more broadly, there is impartiality. Disease does not hit all equally. Certain genetic makeups prevalent in subset populations may make individuals more prone and vulnerable to symptoms and conditions. Different medical conditions may make different populations more susceptible to infections based on their area of residence, workplace environments, or climate of geographical locations. An important relationship to understand is that of socioeconomic status and susceptibility. The idea here is simple, unfortunate, and backed up very seriously by current literature. The idea is that those from lower socioeconomic backgrounds lead less healthy lives, have poorer access to healthcare, diagnostic tests, treatment options, and so, populations concentrated with individuals of relatively lower socioeconomic status experience harder devastations in the face of pandemics and otherwise abnormal environmental conditions.

Chapter 9: Fear and Hysteria around COVID 19

The drastic change in lifestyle caused by COVID-19 has thrown the world into a frenzy. The global unrest has led to almost every major city in the world having an anti-mask protest. Others fear that the restrictions caused by the virus will have a devastating effect on the economy (Klug, 2020). During its inception into the global sphere, so much information was being released about the virus that it became overwhelming for most people. What are we supposed to believe? Who was a reliable source of news? People became fearful. They were scared for their own lives, their children, their friends and loved ones. Moreover, where were they supposed to get their information about the virus? The hysteria seems to have risen immensely from the use of social media. Some of the fears are legitimate. But others seem to have formed from a global panic in which false news relating to the effects and reach of the virus are exaggerated. This panic was only worsened even further by an almost global lockdown which negatively affected mental health at large scale levels. It has made one's perspective on the virus a political view. This chapter will explore the fears related to COVID-19 as well as the related hysteria which has also formed.

Reopening Schools

Let us begin by discussing some of the unanswered fears that COVID-19 has brought about. The novelty of the virus has led to several questions relating to its potency. So far, there is no vaccine and the virus spreads through contact with the infected. This coupled with the closing of schools across the globe, the destruction of the global economy and the flood of social media related fake news has led to a great many fears. Some of these are justified because we simply do not know what is going to happen. In Alberta, the government has opted to open schools in the fall of 2020 (Zakreski, 2020) . This means that teachers will be exposed to 100s of children who may not necessarily know better to wash their hands or wear their face masks all the time. Not only does this likely mean a rise in the number of cases despite the governments' plans. These plans include a great deal of measures such as frequent cleanings, large hand sanitizers at entrances and planning for physical distancing within classrooms. But the issue is that these plans do not account for human behavior. Moreover, they place more work on the already heavy burden which teachers carry in terms of organization. Furthermore, one mistake could lead to a high-risk student or teacher being placed in harm's way. But there is not all bad news for Alberta's schools. If parents decide not to send their kids back in the fall the government will "respect that choice". However, this still does not mitigate the risks posed for teachers (Zakreski, 2020).

To give an example of this idea, I will pull from a CBC interview with an elderly teacher who is considered high risk in Saskatchewan. Her name is Jennifer Gallalys and she suffers from "a respiratory health concern" in the form of severe asthma (Zakreski, 2020) . She is fearful to go back to school and hopes that summer lasts forever. Yet, her life is placed on the backburner to resume "normal life". The information provided so far does not provide any aid to her discomfort with the reopening of schools. Moreover, it makes assumptions about the ability of each school to be able to control the reopening of schools—which it becomes clear to see why it is unjust.

This fear of the virus for teachers extends beyond the Canadian border. In the US, teachers from more than 35 school districts have been protesting over the "plans to resume in-class instruction". The nation is employing similar standards as Alberta but regardless in the country cases are at an all time high with over 4.8 million (O'Brien, 2020) . The country has seen more than 155,000 deaths so far regardless of weak lockdown procedures (O'Brien, 2020). Yet, leaders seem more focused on opening schools than protecting lives.

Economic Impact

Now I will discuss the economic impacts which the virus has created. According to the bank of Canada, the travel, entertainment, and food sectors were those that were affected the most. This comes with little surprise as restaurants, theatres and travel restrictions have led to an almost overnight shutdown of al these industries. The virus also impacted any services which required "face-to-face" communication ("COVID-19", 2020). These include places such as hair salons and dental offices. The fears have led to a large majority of income being removed from people's lives. This in turn, has led to widespread fears about what the economy will look like in the coming year. This reduction of jobs has disproportionately affected women who are more statistically likely to work in affected fields. It is estimated that within the month of March around 1 million Canadians had lost their jobs ("COVID-19", 2020).

The US has seen an even larger decline in employment. Within the first 5 weeks of the virus' impact in the United States, 26 million Americans lost their jobs (Klug, 2020). This has led to a rise in individuals claiming unemployment benefits. The rate eventually rose to 47 million jobs lost at unemployability reaching the Great Depression at 32% (Klug, 2020). The study done by CNBC offers that 67 million US citizens are at high risk of losing their jobs because of the global economy's decline as well. Because of the scope of the virus, it has decimated almost every industry (Klug, 2020).

What this has resulted in, is mass scale protest against the government restrictions in various countries. For example, in Berlin thousands gathered chanting phrases such as "End the corona panic—bring fundamental rights back" (Press, 2020). They believe the government is restricting their freedom due to the virus. They refuse to accept the thousands of people who have died as a result of the virus. In their view, the government is blowing things out of proportion and impeding people's rights (Press, 2020). This all comes because of a hysteria which has resulted because of the virus. They are refusing the facts. Similar protests are taking place all over the world. In Scotland a group called Scotland Against Lockdown has had protests in Scotland with signs truthfully claiming "End Lockdown POVERTY KILLS more than 1%" (Press, 2020). Yet, this group does not look at the broader picture and the increased number of people who would die if the virus spreads more than the comparatively small population which it affects now.

Conspiracy Theories

A previous chapter discussed the rise of fake news in relation to eugenics.

However, it did not discuss its relationship to fear. Moreover, mass scale protests such as those that were discussed previously which occurred in Berlin. Others occurred in Montreal where a crowd protested the Quebec governor who made it mandatory to wear masks in indoor public spaces (Cooke, 2020). Similar policies have taken place all over the world. The mindset of these individuals is that freedom is related to not wearing a mask. These types of protests come from a large spread of misinformation which comes from social media outlets. These types of conspiracy theories are on the rise as well. These lead to devastating consequences which have long term impacts in terms of what COVID-19 is and how it is spread. One study found that misinformation presented on social media is more likely to be believed. And with 16th percent of the Canadian population getting their news from social media websites it becomes easy to see why people are so scared of the false possibility of COVID-19 being some sort of government hoax (Cooke, 2020).

The study which was referenced analyzed 2,500 people through 620,000 tweets. While the political science researcher offered that the false news spreads through other forms of social media such as "Facebook, YouTube, Reddit, Instagram and Tumblr". To highlight other examples of this spread of false news the researcher cited a Facebook group called "Against mandatory mask-wearing in Quebec". The group has over 22,000 followers with similar groups boasting similar numbers (Kestler-D'Amours, 2020). While we previously discussed the hoax that the virus was made in a Chinese lab, other conspiracy theories have risen because of the fear. Other conspiracies include the virus being a way to cover up the effects of 5G technology, hydroxychloroquine being used to cure COVID-19 as well as using saline solution to protect oneself from the virus (Kestler-D'Amours, 2020). Almost half of Canadians believe one of the false conspiracy theories related to COVID-19. It becomes difficult to pinpoint the source of these ideas and the element of fear is a big comparison point to the anti-vaccination movement. Both spread from false news and stem from a sense of fear. Yet, Facebook and other social media platforms are doing their part to remove the fake news from their websites. They routinely remove videos and posts related to the conspiracy theories which were listed. But, that is not enough during these troubling times to mitigate the risks which are being created from the false information (Kestler-D'Amours, 2020). Meek offered that the platform still needs to do more to make sure that people know that the information that they are receiving is false.

The fears largely extend to individual rights. 65-year-old Montreal native Antonio Pietronio offered that the pandemic was "bogus" (Kestler-D'Amours, 2020). His fallacious reasoning assumes that wearing masks will lead the government to force vaccinations against the virus. The people set in this mindset believe the government is just trying to control them. Further offering similarities to the anti-vaccination movement. Alison Meek, a history professor at Western University offered that these individuals are looking for someone to blame because of their fear (Kestler-D'Amours, 2020). The Chinese government and their own government are the easiest targets for it because they are such a large group. There is a lack of trust for the scientific process coupled with anger against lockdown precures has led to public outrage which while unjustified can be understood through the perception of fear. It is likely that this fear of the virus and its related consequences will continue until we have a vaccine on our hands. However, these protests and people refusing to wear the masks will only increase the number of people who are infected leading to more and more deaths.

Conclusion

Chapter 10 & 11: Stereotypes, Misconstructions, and Propaganda
The COVID-19 virus has drastically changed our lives as we know them. We have been forced to alter our way of life in order to minimize the risk to ourselves and those who are in critical conditions. This has led to the creation of conspiracy theories aimed to fill in the blanks of information about the virus that we do not have yet. But, some of these theories are dangerous. They pose a threat to society by undermining the structure that we have set up in order to combat the virus. They see the issue as not the "Virus vs. the People" but rather the "the People vs. the Government". This issue has been exasperated by social media platforms such as Twitter and Facebook. It is understandable that people have fear on the subject. But what some people are doing is irrational and irresponsible because not only does it harm their own lives but also the lives of others.

Chapter 10 & 11: Stereotypes, Misconstructions, and Propaganda

Covid-19 has placed a lasting impact on everybody in society and the way we operate. Whether it be jobs, mindsets, social practices, etc, we have changed. Along with Covid-19, there has also been a surge of stereotypes, misconceptions, and propaganda curated by society to influence and trap certain members for their own gain.

Stereotypes and Covid-19

Stereotypes impact the way that we view society, they are the product of what we believe after all. They are the characters that we make up in our heads and assign any person who loosely fits the cut to be that personality. They are often not true and allow us to judge people without knowing anything about them. Covid-19 has introduced varying stereotypes to the world and they are extremely common for us to believe in them when we hear about someone on the news or see someone in person. These stereotypes have impacted so many individuals and boxed them into something that they may not be, we have placed labels and tags on people that are not true.

The Affected Asian

This is basically any Asian that you see, really. Any asian looking human being, East-Asian to be specific, is boxed into this character. So they are the ones that have apparently brought the virus to every country on the globe, and they are responsible for the virus in general. The virus was called the "Chinese Virus" by even Donald Trump, only reinforcing this character even more. Every time they leave their house, they get stares and comments that suggest that they need to 'take their virus back to their country'. Do these asians actually have anything to do with the making of Covid-19 at all? No, but the virus started in Wuhan, China, so now every East-Asian is responsible. They are apparently carriers of the virus as well, so people make sure to stay away from them in public and make in be known that they are the sole and root cause. Chinese, Japanese, Taiwanese, Korean, Mogolian, etc, they all fit the bill. If someone looks visibly East-Asian or could pass as one, guess what, they apparently have the virus.

The Wildchild

The teenager that you see in the mall, park, or anywhere to be honest, if they are outside, this is them. The wildchild is someone who does not care about health measures that come with the virus at all, they do their own thing. They are rebellious youngsters who do as they please, and don't care for themselves or the people that surround them. They hate that they can't hang out with friends, and because of this, they will. As long as they don't get into trouble with the law, the world is their pickle. These teenagers are the ones who are not allowing the virus to be contained and are responsible for the spread and new cases everyday. Some have even began 'Covid Parties' in which the first to get the virus from their friend group receives a prize. They have made the virus into a joke, not thinking about how it is the cause of death for many people around the world. So, are all teenagers like this? Definitely not, but most of them are seen as 'The Wildchild' because they are young.

The Responsible Middle-Aged

The middle-aged man or woman who is doing their part, and doing it amazingly. They are following every health and safety measure put into place and actively doing their part to limit the spread of the virus. They are taking care of not only themselves, but their parents and children as well. The 'Responsible Middle-Aged' person looks like, well a middle-aged person. Slightly older, probably will have graying hair, and the signs of aging have begun to show on their face. They go to work, safely, and ensure that they are being careful and not doing anything that they should not be doing. They go for groceries, and other only essential errands, and there they are wearing a mask, keeping their distance from other customers, sanitizing regularly, and might even be wearing gloves. These are the people that also get groceries for their parents or any elderly in their neighbourhood, making sure to sanitize the products before giving them. They are essentially the model citizens that we should all be following their example to limit the spread and demolish the virus. The thing is that not every middle-aged person is exactly responsible like this, some may be, most might be actually. But not every single middle-aged human is 'The Responsible Middle-Aged'.

The MAGA Enthusiast

Your typical racist, white supremacist, and dumb citizen. These are the people who are Trump supporters or sympathizers more often than not and act as if they know everything that there is to know about the virus. These are also the same people who believe that chocolate milk comes from brown cows and that the Earth is indeed flat. They spread fake news on the daily and have that 'Texas' aura about them. Some choose not to wear a mask as much as possible because they believe that is has something to do about politics and not actual safety, it's all a scheme according to them. Trump made a comment abut injecting disinfectant into citizens to eradicate the virus, and The MAGA Enthusiast actually took his words seriously. This person is the one who actually did try to ingest disinfectants to eradicate the virus, they might not be the most well-informed in the world. They are also the people who still have gatherings exceeding the limits as much as they can because again, the virus is government lies to them and they have nothing to fear. Not every white person is automatically this character and as clueless or racist as they are painted. Some most certainly are like this, but not everyone is.

The Exposed Elderly

It is known that the elderly and people with immune issues are the most effected by Covid-19, but as the virus. This is where The Exposed Elderly kicks in, they are the ones that you hardly see outside. They are vulnerable and need to protected, their social lives or mental wellbeing don't really matter in this case. They are old, so they need to stay at home, they have no reason to leave the house because their children or someone else can run their errands. If you want to visit an Exposed Elderly, you need to be thoroughly sanitized and ensure that there is absolutely a zero percent chance that you have the virus or have come into contact with it, which does make sense. Often, it is forgotten that even though the elderly may be vulnerable, they have lives as well. We cannot isolate them completely, and not every single elderly is as vulnerable or effected as we may think. There are ways to ensure that they are staying safe and still living a satisfying life at the same time.

Covid-19 is a virus that we learn something new about almost everyday. There is much that we still don't know and are trying our best to understand and grasp exactly what it is and how we can combat it. Developing vaccines is one of our main priorities and also helping the patients that are already sick heal and recover. Due to the fact that Covid-19 is as hazy as it is, people are trying their best to make sense of it and believing whatever they hear. People reinforce random information and facts that they hear about from friends, family, and websites. People believe any sort of misconstructions or propaganda that they hear so that they know something at least. In a time of uncertainty, people want to grasp onto any information that they can so that they can feel somewhat in control.

Trump and Disinfectants

One common misconstruction and form of propaganda is when Donald Trump suggested that using a disinfectant could have potential to cure Covid-19. He later claimed that he was only being sarcastic and joking, but this left an impact on people who heard about this event. Many people did indeed try and ingested disinfectants for the sake of the virus. Clorox even had to issue a statement warning individuals against ingesting an of their products. This is an example of a misconstruction that misled many people and caused them to do acts that were harmful and potentially deadly to their lives.

Covid-19 a Hoax or Government Lies

Some people believe in the fact that Covid-19 is a hoax. This is something that many accepted and said that it was all just an elaborate scheme that health officials and various governments curated. The logistics behind this wild misconstruction is non-existent, but people tend to believe what is the most convenient for them. Many are scared and want to believe that the virus is false and cannot effect them, as outrageous as it may seem. Other theories surrounding the validity of Covid-19 have also emerged such as the severity of it and the numbers are fake. This is also simply just a form of misconstruction and people choosing to believe untrustworthy posts that they see online. When these individuals begin to trust in these pieces of information, they start to disregard the virus and don't follow the safety precautions that they must. This contributes to the spread of the virus, and at that rate, we will never fully rid ourselves of it.

Pepper as a Covid-19 Prevention/Cure

A piece of information going around was that pepper somehow helped cure or prevent Covid-19, which is false. Misconstructions like this spread from people seeing and sharing these kinds of posts of Facebook or Instagram. People then begin to believe them and start acting on them, in hopes that it will save them from the virus. People began putting a large amount of pepper in their soups and meals, thinking that it would help them in prevention or even in curing the virus. This was a misconstruction that fooled people and wasted their time and energy.

Covid-19 has influenced all members of society and their way of life. We have begun to live in a different way and have even adopted some new beliefs and values. Covid-19 has introduced many stereotypes, misconceptions, and propaganda which has shaped these new beliefs and values. We need to steer clear of the negative aspects of these stereotypes, misconceptions, and propaganda in order to stay educated and protect ourselves and society so that we can stop the virus.

Chapter 12: Vulnerability and Anxieties

Covid-19 is a pandemic, and with a pandemic comes obstacles to the economy, society, and individuals. A consequence to Covid-19, and other pandemics in general, is the vulnerability and anxieties that individuals begin to experience.

Anxiety and Covid-19

Anxiety, according to the Oxford Languages, is "a feeling of worry, nervousness, or unease, typically about an imminent event or something with an uncertain outcome." This fear is common among many individuals, however, Covid-19 is a key player in influencing these numbers recently. With the rise of Covid-19, anxiety levels in individuals have also spiked, (1).

Quarantine and Social Distancing

Covid-19 has a huge role in introducing anxiety and fear within individuals, and for good reason too. Nobody is certain about the outcome of the virus, and it can affect anybody and everybody. People are scared of losing their loved ones and themselves to this deadly virus and no one is immune. However, as the government is trying to minimize the spread and effects of COVID, quarantine and self-isolation practices have been put into place and with these to come consequences. Isolation from loved ones, friends, and family add to this anxiety. In times of discomfort and uncertainty, people turn to those closest to them to seek solace and comfort, but when they are unable to do this, they begin to feel helpless. It is crucial to have a support system when you lose your confidence and begin to fall into a dark place, but due to Covid-19, for so many, this is not possible. Social distancing also contributes to this anxiety because not being able to be near human contact, even friends and family aside, can have a detrimental effect on your anxiety. You are not able to go to enjoy the mall, go bowling, watch a movie, or do anything that normally relieves stress for you. Being stuck at home with no outlets or people to relieve your stress and fears can be extremely hard and increase your anxiety levels by a large margin. As boredom and loneliness increase, it is guaranteed that people develop more fear and their pre-existing mental health conditions can weaken.

Anxiety and Pre-existing Mental Illness

Anxiety is not an illness that was introduced with Covid-19, it was always existing. However, the virus and public health measures that have been put into place to reduce the spread have effected those who already suffer from anxiety. With the news, social media posts, and general discussion of the virus, people who have issues with fear and discomfort experience it even more. The virus serves as another source of uncertainty for anxiety patients and gives them one more stress to take into account. People begin to question whether or not they will ever be able to live in and contribute to society the way that they were able to in the past. Will they survive? Will their parents survive? Will we ever find a vaccine? These are all thoughts and concerns that can plague the mind and make it difficult for those who already struggle with staying positive even more. In addition to this, the effects of the virus also contribute to depressions and mental illness in general. Some who may have had severe anxiety before the pandemic is susceptible to depression developing with the overwhelming amount of darkness now shrouding their life.

Covid-19 has interfered with pre-existing anxiety and has not allowed for individuals to seek help as even offices are closed. For those who actively wish to improve their anxiety and speak to someone professional who can help them sort out their thoughts, they need to visit a therapist. It has become complicated to reach out to professionals at this time, and even though things are slowly opening up, some may not wish to go through this elaborate process to speak to someone. They now need to wear a mask and practice social distancing, which to some is not worth the effort. In addition to this, the cases are not decreasing and a lot of people fear to catch the virus by stepping outside of their houses. Reaching out via calls and text is still available, however, even this isn't a simple and convenient process and again, some would not go through the effort. Many individuals may not feel comfortable talking over the phone and sharing themselves if it is not in a physical setting. There are countless ways in which how Covid-19 has impacted one's anxiety, pre-existing anxieties, and hasn't allowed for an individual to fully seek adequate help.

Consequences of Anxiety and Covid-19

It is apparent that Covid-19 has a direct link to anxiety and has helped shape the way society feels operates. With this anxiety, there are some consequences to individuals and society that arise and pose as another difficulty in this already difficult period. When the stress and fears begin to accumulate, they can lead to individuals taking extreme measures to subdue their discomfort. If one has anxiety about ever leaving the house, they may begin to over-purchase groceries and supplies that are needed for everybody, (3). A specific example would be gloves, masks, or hand sanitizers, for someone who severely fears to come into contact with the virus. This person may buy in bulk, and if there are no restrictions on buying, this will impact the supply for those who need it urgently. Another effect of this increase od anxiety with be denial, (3). This is when people refuse to believe that the virus can impact them or refuse to take any safety precautions to help them. This can severely impact the spread of the virus because if people refuse to take it seriously, the spread can never decrease. It puts all of the country's efforts to control the virus to risk and if people are not making an effort to help, the virus will not end. Despite the ever-growing anxiety, there are methods that one can take to minimize their anxiety and try to gain a more positive outlook on life.

Solutions to avoid this anxiety

There are lifestyle improvements and even little improvements that can be taken to help reduce this anxiety and the consequences that come along with it.

Taking Action: One thing that can be done is taking action. This includes reading up on the virus and seeing how you can limit the spread. Follow trusted government sites to be informed on how you can be kept safe and do your part. (3). This will ensure that as much as uncertainty and fear can be erased from your mind as possible, the more you know, the more confident and secure you feel about yourself.

Attending to Yourself: Another step that can be taken in ensuring that you are attending to yourself. This includes forcing yourself to sleep well, eat well, and engaging in any hobbies or interests that you have. You can even explore different stress-relieving activities that can help with tension such as yoga or art. (3) You need to maintain your health and force yourself to keep busy as a distraction and stress-reliever.

Stay Connected: Staying connected means that you are still reaching out to your family and friends, even if it is just by texting and calling. This also means that you are connected with those who need your help, and you are helping out others if you can in terms of supplies or even just emotional support. Staying connected also involves seeking out any help if you are struggling despite all of your efforts and need further help. You can contact a professional call different hotlines, or visit websites that are now available for Covid-19 assistance. (3).

As diseases and illnesses spread, particular individuals are especially vulnerable, mental vulnerabilities include the increase of anxiety and anxiety-related issues, but some are physically vulnerable as well.

Vulnerability and Covid-19

As diseases and illnesses spread, particular individuals are especially vulnerable to catching them, and this puts their life in jeopardy, (2). Those populations who may acquire Covid-19 faster than others or have more severe symptoms require extra care and assistance to ensure their safety.

Those Who are Vulnerable

People who are the elderly, have pre-existing medical conditions or have a compromised immune system from medical treatments or conditions (2). People who have difficulties with basic literature and communication skills, have difficulties obtaining medical advice and healthcare, have difficulties taking the public health measures, have specialized medical and non-medical needs, have no access to transportation, have economic difficulties, have difficulties within their working place or conditions, live in a geographically isolated area, or have no satisfactory housing. (2).

How the Vulnerable Populations can be Supported

Inform: Something that all individuals can do to help out the vulnerable populations is by informing. This includes doing anything you can to inform and instruct the vulnerable populations that you can reach. If you speak their language, teach them how to wash their hands, to put on maks, to practice social distancing, etc. You can create blogs, make posters, hang up signs, and much more. Do whatever you can to help out and teach whatever you know to those who have difficulties doing so on their own. (2)

Provide Support: Providing support is another way in which we can help out the vulnerable. This can be done in small gestures or large ones. This involves helping out, if you can, by providing housing, medications, or transportation to those who need it, (2). This ensures that those who need extra resources to maintain their living receive it and are not deprived based on complications that are not in their hands. Everybody has different resources so what you can do to support is dependant on you, but anything at all helps.

A pandemic causes many different complications and difficulties to the society and members of the society as well. People can develop anxiety and this leads to other complications, but there are ways to control this anxiety if an effort is put into it. Mental vulnerabilities are not the only ones present, and there are physical ones as well. Certain populations are more vulnerable to the virus than others and there are measures that we can take to help them maintain a healthy life. Amidst the chaos and mayhem that Covid-19 has caused and will continue to cause, there are different steps that we can take to help ourselves and those around us so that we can get through this troubling period.

Chapter 13: Preventing Hate Crime

Hate Crime impacts everybody in society. Hate crime is a cycle, an infectious one that is. In that, it must be dealt with caution and eliminated as witnessed. For a safe society to grow, the causative agents of hate crime must be attended to first—hate crime must be prevented. Preventing hate crime is a step necessary for the productivity of society, a stepping stone for improvements in the quality of life of all members of a community.

Why Prevent Hate Crime?

In a world where every individual is granted legal rights and equality, everyone deserves to be treated with at least basic human decency. Safety and security is the bare minimum all deserve. Yet, hate crime threatens just that. Hate crime threatens individuals through physical, mental, or emotional harm. Although the most common type of hate crime involves assault, hate crime usually includes harm extending over multiple areas of concern.

Stabbings, shootings, running people over with vehicles, hitting, pushing, and more are all the kinds of experiences that a person goes through when they are targeted for their race. It is obvious that this is extremely negative and that nobody should have to be a victim of any sort of bodily harm, which is purely a result of how they look or what they choose to stand for. It is a violation of them, their rights, their beliefs, and their character.

It is often seen that these physical attacks not only hurt a person just physically- they lead to other mental and emotional challenges. When someone is attacked out of spite and hate, they begin to struggle with

identity and self-acceptance. This impacts their life and allows them to feel unnecessarily endangered in their environment. These people begin to lose the sense of community and belonging that they may have felt and start fearing for their lives on the daily. Mental and emotional side-effects also plague those who are a part of the community that a Hate Crime has taken place against. Countless Arab students fled back home after the September 11 attacks in America. These individuals did nothing except sharing the same race as a group of terrorists. However, after witnessing so much hate and negativity against them, they left. The hate surely left a lasting impact on their mental and emotional health and left a very obvious impact on how they viewed their position in society.

Hate Crime is like the flu, without a vaccine ever forming or being applied, it is impossible to prevent. It spreads to all households and becomes common. Hate Crime must be prevented, and if not, it will become normalized and contribute to a toxic environment. In a place where Hate Crime is usual, people will stop functioning as an effective community, because many are scared and unwilling to risk themselves to participate out of fear of retaliation from the perpetrators. In order for populations to operate smoothly, they demand to depend on each other and exchange services. If Hate Crime is present, this dependency begins to diminish and the community is no longer cohesive and successful. Hate Crime impacts society as a whole and as individuals, which is why it needs to be prevented.

How to Prevent Hate Crime

Take Action:

If we do not take action against the Hate Crime that is expanding in our communities, it will accumulate and spread. The first and foremost step in taking a stance to prevent Hate Crime from occurring is acting. We must take action as opposed to quietly condemning it in our hearts, as there is no benefit to this and it may be seen as acceptance. The hate is harming not only the victims but the community as it causes division and separation between ethnic groups. If Hate Crime is not stopped in its earlier stages, it can heighten from verbal harassment to even physical violence, which is why we need to act against it. Some ways that you can act against Hate Crime are beginning to bring up the conversation to your loved ones and friends, start suggesting some action in any way you can. You can sign petitions, attend peaceful rallies, go to vigils, help remove racist vandalism, create pamphlets, and so on. The list is endless and every individual has different abilities, restrictions, and skills so what you do is generally unique to you.

Create a Community:

Just like yourself, there are dozens and hundreds of individuals in each community that do not stand for Hate Crime. Many people are waiting for a cause, organization, or anything really that they can turn to show their support. Many are also afraid and scared to speak out against Hate Crime. Whatever the case, people need an organized and comfortable place to turn to plan against preventing Hate Crime. This is why it is crucial for you to reach out and create a community. There is strength in numbers, and not only does a community erase the fear that often is associated with speaking out against injustice, but it also creates new channels of creativity and collaboration. It is far easier to create ideas and projects in a team, and creating a community allows for this. When the community is united, you can begin to educate those around you about Hate Crime and even start forming a healthy relationship with the law enforcers. To create a community, what you can do is invite groups and organizations that are expected to react to Hate Crime. These groups can be in universities, councils, charities, schools, businesses, and so on. Any group that you believe will stand against Hate Crime so that we can prevent it in the future, you can communicate to.

Assist the Victims:

Often times, victims of Hate Crime feel alone and isolated. They feel like they were targeted for a reason and begin to feel like nobody in the community cares for them. This is why, when you learn about a Hate Crime that takes place in your area, showing support to the victims is key. You need to let them know that you stand with them and that they are not alone. This helps in preventing Hate Crime because it shows the perpetrators that the victims have support and are not alone, preventing similar cases from taking place in the future. Your support is a symbol of unity, and an army of people is less likely to be sought out for hate as opposed to one individual. By lending your kindness, other victims may also feel encouraged to step up and report incidents, and this will help

74

with the overall number of Hate Crimes decreasing. If you are a victim yourself, what you can do is report every hateful incident to the police, get media coverage so that other victims may feel less alone, research your rights as a human being, support other victims, and so on. You, whether you are a victim or supporter, can do so much to help other victims and this in the long run can help prevent Hate Crime.

Use your Voice

Use your voice to prevent hate crime, speak up. This is when you need to be public and work hand in hand with the media to get coverage and spread awareness on Hate Crimes. It is important to speak out against Hate Crime and tell the victims stories. Doing this scares the perpetrators from acting out again when they see how much coverage and bad recognition their actions are receiving. However, fighting with hate activists is not an ideal way to use your voice, instead, turn to other and more effective ways to spread your message. You can hand out posters, attend debates, go to radio shows, go to news shows, write articles, start blogs, etc. You can do anything that you know will help in the prevention of hate crime by using public awareness and the media. Your voice is one of the most powerful tools and using it for good helps the entire community.

Educate Yourself:

As an individual passionate about preventing Hate Crime, so that the spread and negative effects of it can become limited, there are many things that can be done. Often times, it is difficult for individuals to help in the prevention of Hate Crime solely due to their ignorance. Many people are unable to take a stance against Hate Crime because they are unaware that it even takes place in the first place. This is why a way that you can aid in the prevention of Hate Crime is by educating yourself. Research and track cases of Hate Crimes that have taken place in your area so that you can later take action against them. Be familiar with the terms and history of Hate Crime and which groups have been targeted. Study and become familiarized with anything and everything that you can so that once you have become knowledgeable, the next step that you can take is teaching others. The only way that Hate Crime can be prevented is if people are aware that it is taking place in the first place. You must do whatever you can -no amount is too little- to first educate yourself and then educate others on what Hate Crime is, who it affects, and why it is wrong. By doing this, you are uncovering another layer in preventing Hate Crime.

Give a Positive Cause

Often times in the face of Hate Crime, it is extremely tempting to fight back and engage with the perpetrators and their supporters. However, it is imperative that as an activist who wishes to end Hate Crime, you must give the people a positive cause instead. Instead of fighting and bashing the racists, you can begin peaceful protests. There are numerous positive outlets to pursue instead of turning to hate and evil. You should avoid all forms of hate-fueled events and instead create peaceful situations for individuals so that they don't fear for their security and safety. Fighting fire with fire only ever results in added fire, and your purpose is to end this hate, to douse the fire and not add to it. There is a lot of passion and enthusiasm that erupts when hate is presented, but with your help and productive plans, this passion can be channeled to do something that can actually make a change. You and your community can construct a vision that can aid in the prevention of Hate Crime, and not engage with the hate when you know there is no positive outcome.

Advertise Acceptance:

An issue with hate and Hate Crimes is that they begin from somewhere. One doesn't just wake up one day and decide to punish a person based on their appearance, religion, sexuality, etc., they allowed the ideas to brew. A major method of preventing Hate Crimes is by promoting and advertising acceptance everywhere and at every time. Racist jokes, racist slurs, inclusivity, and all forms of disdain towards a group of individuals need to be destroyed. Hate Crimes start from less extreme actions such as thoughts and feelings towards someone, if this can be prevented then so can Hate Crimes. Advertise acceptance by visiting schools and teaching young children the importance of exclusivity, go to universities and colleges, advertise in your workplace, etc. You can make a difference everywhere, even at home! Teach your children, siblings or parents to remove any biases that they may have. You can display acceptance in your everyday behaviour and tone, set an example for those around you.

Hate Crime is not something to take lightly. If we do not speak out and address it, it will only escalate and accumulate. Work on yourself and those around you for the betterment of your community, and ultimately the world.

Chapter 14: Conclusion

The COVID-19 pandemic has been life-changing for us all. People are in fear of the unknown, of their safety, and recovery. Businesses have their own worries, countries their own measures to set, modify, and attend to. Scientists, medical professionals, and public health workers collaborate to better understand the pathophysiology of the novel virus. In fact, we all connect in our curiosity, discussion, and optimism or lack thereof for "flattening the curve." Indeed, we are all collaborators. The shared substance affirms the idea that nothing in this pandemic happens in isolation, there are sociological factors, variables, and influences that affect every aspect of the pandemic. Racism and hate crimes are but one of the shaping forces of the pandemic. Nonetheless, the COVID-19 pandemic has been heavily racialized. One could study medicinal history, biowarfare and eugenics, or delve into the history of hate crimes against ethnic groups, other cases of racialized diseases such as the Holocaust and SARS, and begin to realize how linked race and disease have been established as. There are demographics and socioeconomic distribution of disease. The COVID-19 pandemic, in particular, presented an alarming incidence of hate crimes against Asians, as well as racist language coined. Stereotypes were reinforced, and misconstructions and propaganda spread throughout the pandemic. In these cases, there are emotions involved on both sides, there is fear and hysteria, for example. There is also vulnerability and anxieties involved.

In studying these factors, it is pivotal to keep the prevention of hate crime at a priority. Hate Crime is fully preventable if we make conscious efforts to educate ourselves and help reinforce the law and universal laws of goodness. Each step we take makes a difference in progressing towards a more ideal state of society, where everyone feels safe and comfortable in their skin and environment. The more we let it slide, the worse situations will get. It takes each of us to do something, as a matter of fact, it is our responsibility as goodwill ambassadors and active global citizens to do what it takes to address the racialization and hate crimes, especially in this dire time.

Bibliography

Covid-19 Fueling Anti-Asian Racism and Xenophobia Worldwide. (2020, August 08). Retrieved August 09, 2020, from https://www. hrw.org/news/2020/05/12/covid-19-fueling-anti-asian-racism-and-xenophobia-worldwide

Foster, L. (2006, July/August). The Process of "Racialization". Retrieved August 09, 2020, from http://www.yorku.ca/ lfoster/2006-07/sosi4440b/lectures/RACIALIZATION_ THEPROCESSOFRACIALIZATION.html

Heshmat, S. (2015, April 23). What Is Confirmation Bias? Retrieved August 09, 2020, from https://www.psychologytoday.com/ca/ blog/science-choice/201504/what-is-confirmation-bias

Kang, P. (2020, April 16). What it means to be Asian during COVID-19. Retrieved August 09, 2020, from https://www.thestar.com/ opinion/contributors/2020/04/16/what-it-means-to-be-asian-during-covid-19.html

Understanding the impact of COVID-19 on the Asian community. (n.d.). Retrieved August 09, 2020, from http://psacunion.ca/ understanding-impact-covid-19-asian-community

(n.d.). Q&A on coronaviruses (COVID-19). Retrieved August 09, 2020, from https://www.who.int/emergencies/diseases/novel-coronavirus-2019/question-and-answers-hub/q-a-detail/q-a-coronaviruses

Carbonaro, G. (2020, May 23). Is COVID-19 a bioweapon? Here's what the experts say. Retrieved July 21, 2020, from https://newseu.cgtn. com/news/2020-05-23/Is-COVID-19-a-bioweapon-Here-s-what-the-experts-say-QHUXqEGDVC/index.html

Dodds, C., & Karlsen, S. (2020, May 30). Ethnicity and Covid-19: Standing on the shoulders of eugenics?. https://doi.org/10.31235/osf.io/5gbrz

Graham, R. (2020, May 25). Eugenics and the White Moderate: Reflections on the COVID Crisis from Reconstruction (Guest Post). Retrieved July 21, 2020, from https://s-usih.org/2020/05/eugenics-and-the-white-moderate-reflections-on-the-covid-crisis-from-reconstruction-guest-post/

Heil, E., & Carman, T. (2020, February 14). Amid coronavirus fears, Chinese restaurants report a drop in business. Retrieved August 11, 2020, from https://www.washingtonpost.com/lifestyle/food/amid-coronavirus-fears-chinese-restaurants-report-a-drop-in-business/2020/02/14/2c7d7efe-4e8f-11ea-bf44-f5043eb3918a_story.html

Jones, S. (2020, March 25). Eugenics Isn't Going to Get Us Out of This Mess. Retrieved July 21, 2020, from https://nymag.com/intelligencer/2020/03/eugenics-isnt-going-to-save-you-from-coronavirus.html

Jones, S. (2020, January 02). Will the 2020s Be the Decade of Eugenics? Retrieved July 21, 2020, from https://nymag.com/intelligencer/2020/01/eugenic-ideas-never-really-went-away.html

Kaszeta, D. (2020, April 27). Perspective | No, the coronavirus is not a biological weapon. Retrieved July 21, 2020, from https://www.washingtonpost.com/outlook/2020/04/26/no-coronavirus-is-not-biological-weapon/

Lee, B. (2020, March 24). No, COVID-19 Coronavirus Was Not Bioengineered. Here's The Research That Debunks That Idea. Retrieved July 21, 2020, from https://www.forbes.com/sites/brucelee/2020/03/17/covid-19-coronavirus-did-not-come-from-a-lab-study-shows-natural-origins/

Shanks, P. (2020, May/June). Confronting Racist Eugenics in the Pandemic. Retrieved July 21, 2020, from https://www.geneticsandsociety.org/biopolitical-times/confronting-racist-eugenics-pandemic

Ahrens, D., Aoki, K., Barde, R., J. Burton, M., Chen, T., Chin, G., . . . Zheng, B. (2020, July 07). Anti-Asian Hate Crime During the

COVID-19 Pandemic: Exploring the Reproduction of Inequality. Retrieved July 31, 2020, from https://link.springer.com/article/10.1007/s12103-020-09545-1

Astor, M. (2018, April 12). Holocaust Is Fading From Memory, Survey Finds. Retrieved July 31, 2020, from https://www.nytimes.com/2018/04/12/us/holocaust-education.html

Iturralde C. (2009), Rhetoric and Violence: Understanding Incidents of Hate Against Latinos, 12 N.Y. City L. Rev. 417. Retrieved July, 31, 2020 Available at: 10.31641/clr120207

Government of Canada, D. (2015, January 07). Disproportionate Harm: Hate Crime in Canada. Retrieved July 31, 2020, from https://www.justice.gc.ca/eng/rp-pr/csj-sjc/crime/wd95_11-dt95_11/p0_1.html

Hassan, A. (2019, November 12). Hate-Crime Violence Hits 16-Year High, F.B.I. Reports. Retrieved July 31, 2020, from https://www.nytimes.com/2019/11/12/us/hate-crimes-fbi-report.html

Halim, F. (2019, April 03). Why do hate crimes against Muslims increase? Retrieved July 31, 2020, from https://leaderpost.com/opinion/columnists/why-do-hate-crimes-against-muslims-increase

History of Lynchings. (2020). Retrieved July 31, 2020, from https://www.naacp.org/history-of-lynchings/

Lartey, J., & Morris, S. (2018, April 26). How white Americans used lynchings to terrorize and control black people. Retrieved July 31, 2020, from https://www.theguardian.com/us-news/2018/apr/26/lynchings-memorial-us-south-montgomery-alabama

Lazarus, D. (2019, July 24). Jews Are The Most Targeted Minority Group In Canada, Study Shows. Retrieved July 31, 2020, from https://forward.com/fast-forward/428174/canada-jews-anti-semitism-hate-crime-police/

Mosley, T. (2019, November 25). The 'Forgotten' History Of Anti-Latino Violence In The U.S. Retrieved July 31, 2020, from https://www.wbur.org/hereandnow/2019/11/25/history-violence-against-latinos

Walters, Q. (2020, May 12). Anti-Semitic Crime In The U.S. Reaches Record Levels. Retrieved July 31, 2020, from https://www.wbur.

org/news/2020/05/12/antisemitic-crime-record-level

Zine, J. (2020, June 09). Islamophobia and hate crimes continue to rise in Canada. Retrieved July 31, 2020, from https://theconversation. com/islamophobia-and-hate-crimes-continue-to-rise-in-canada-110635

DB, S. (1998). Addressing racial inequities in health care: civil rights monitoring and report cards. Health Politics, Policy and Law, 23:75-105.

D'Sa, P. (2020, January 29). SARS-Fuelled Racism Scarred Chinese-Canadians. It's Happening Again With Coronavirus. Retrieved from huffingtonpost.ca: https://www.huffingtonpost.ca/entry/coronavirus-sars-racism-canada_ca_5e3241f6c5b611ac94cf4b36

G, K. (1996). Ethnicity & Disease. In K. G, Institutional racism and the medical/health complex: a conceptual analysis (pp. 6:30-46). PubMed.

G, M. (1944). An American Dilemma Vol 1. New York: Harper & Brothers Publishers.

Geiger, H. (1996). Race and health care-an American dilemma? New England Journal of Medicine, 335:815-816.

H, M. (1999). Distrust, social justice, and health care. Mount Sinai Journal of Medicine, 66:236-240.

Jewish Badges During The Holocaust: Photographs & Overview. (2020, June 20). Retrieved from Jewish Virtual Library: https://www.jewishvirtuallibrary.org/photographs-and-overview-of-jewish-badges-in-the-holocaust

Lee, K. (2013). SARS and Its Reasoning Impact on the Asian Communities. Retrieved from Lehigh Preserve: https://preserve.lehigh.edu/cgi/viewcontent.cgi?article=1015&context=cas-lehighreview-vol-21

Sala, I. M. (2020, February 12). Hong Kong's coronavirus panic buying isn't hysteria, it's unresolved trauma. Retrieved from Quartz: https://qz.com/1798974/how-sars-trauma-made-hong-kong-distrust-beijing/

Stone, L. (2019, January 2). Quantifying the Holocaust: Hyperintense Kill Rates During the Nazi Genocide. Retrieved from Science

Advances: https://advances.sciencemag.org/content/5/1/eaau7292

United States Holocaust Memorial Council. (2020, June 11). Documenting the Numbers of Victims of the holocaust and Nazi Persecution. Retrieved from United States Holocaust Memorial Museum: https://encyclopedia.ushmm.org/content/en/article/documenting-numbers-of-victims-of-the-holocaust-and-nazi-persecution

United States Holocaust Memorial Council. (2020, June 11). Introduction to the Holocaust. Retrieved from United States Holocaust Memorial Museum: https://encyclopedia.ushmm.org/content/en/article/introduction-to-the-holocaust

United States Holocaust Memorial Council. (2020, June 11). Nuremberg Laws. Retrieved from United States Holocaust Memorial Museum: https://encyclopedia.ushmm.org/content/en/article/nuremberg-laws

United States Holocaust Memorial Council. (2020, June 11). The Holocaust and World War II: Key Dates. Retrieved from United States Holocaust Memorial Museum: https://encyclopedia.ushmm.org/content/en/article/the-holocaust-and-world-war-ii-key-dates

Williams DR, R. T. (2000). Understanding and addressing racial disparities in health care. Health Care Financing Review, 21:75-90.

Sirleaf, M. (2020, July 4). COVID-19 Symposium: COVID-19 and the Racialization of Diseases (Part I). Retrieved July 31, 2020, from

http://opiniojuris.org/2020/04/07/covid-19-symposium-covid-19-and-the-racialization-of-diseases-part-i/

Cho, J. (2020, March 10). Coronavirus panic: Media blends elements of "yellow peril" and Red Scare. Retrieved July 31, 2020, from https://www.salon.com/2020/03/10/coronavirus-panic-media-blends-elements-of-yellow-peril-and-red-scare_partner/

Ali, H. and Kurasawa F. (2020, March 22). #COVID19: Social media both a blessing and a curse during coronavirus pandemic. Retrieved July 31, 2020, from

https://theconversation.com/covid19-social-media-both-a-blessing-and-a-curse-during-coronavirus-pandemic-133596

Benefits Canada Staff. (2020, August 6). Index shows coronavirus, response to racism affecting Canadians' mental health. Retrieved July 31, 2020, from

https://www.benefitscanada.com/news/coronavirus-increased-response-to-racism-affecting-canadians-mental-health-survey-148610

Cooke, A. (2020, July 20). Unmasking the dangers of false COVID-19 rhetoric | CBC News. Retrieved August 06, 2020, from https://www.cbc.ca/news/canada/nova-scotia/covid-19-misinformation-conspiracy-theories-1.5655460

COVID-19: Actions to Support the Economy and Financial System. (n.d.). Retrieved August 06, 2020, from https://www.bankofcanada.ca/markets/market-operations-liquidity-provision/covid-19-actions-support-economy-financial-system/

Craven , M., & Liu, L. (2020, July 30). COVID-19: Implications for business. Retrieved August 06, 2020, from https://www.mckinsey.com/business-functions/risk/our-insights/covid-19-implications-for-business

Klug, F. (2020, March 01). COVID-19: Coronavirus outbreak shakes global economy as fear grows. Retrieved August 06, 2020, from https://globalnews.ca/news/6615465/coronavirus-economic-impact/

Kestler-D'Amours, J. (2020, August 03). COVID-19 conspiracy theories creating a 'public health crisis' in Canada, experts say | CBC News. Retrieved August 06, 2020, from https://www.cbc.ca/news/politics/covid-19-conspiracy-theories-1.5672766

O'Brien, B. (2020, August 03). Teachers protest reopening of US schools while coronavirus lurks. Retrieved August 06, 2020, from https://www.smh.com.au/world/north-america/teachers-protest-reopening-of-us-schools-while-coronavirus-lurks-20200804-p55i8j.html

Press, T. (2020, August 01). Thousands protest in Berlin against coronavirus restrictions. Retrieved August 06, 2020, from http://www.ctvnews.ca/health/coronavirus/thousands-protest-in-berlin-against-coronavirus-restrictions-1.5048090

Zakreski, D. (2020, August 03). Teachers grappling with fear and uncertainty as return to the classroom looms | CBC News. Retrieved August 06, 2020, from https://www.cbc.ca/news/canada/saskatoon/teachers-grappling-with-fear-and-uncertainty-as-return-to-the-classroom-looms-1.5670178

Murray, J. and Sherwood H. (2013, March 13). Anxiety on rise due to coronavirus, say mental health charities. Retrieved _____, from

https://www.theguardian.com/world/2020/mar/13/anxiety-on-rise-due-to-coronavirus-say-mental-health-charities

Government of Canada. (2020, July 20). Vulnerable populations and COVID-19. Retrieved _____, from

https://www.canada.ca/en/public-health/services/publications/diseases-conditions/vulnerable-populations-covid-19.html

The Canadian Mental Health Association. (2020). COVID-19 and Anxiety. Retrieved _____, from https://www.heretohelp.bc.ca/infosheet/covid-19-and-anxiety